Crohn's Disease - The Current State of the Art

Edited by Partha Pal

Published in London, United Kingdom

Crohn's Disease - The Current State of the Art
http://dx.doi.org/10.5772/intechopen.104329
Edited by Partha Pal

Contributors
Gulustan H. Babayeva, Gunay V. Asadova, Jamal S. Musayev, Umud R. Mahmudov, Farid V. Quliyev, Aychin I. Hasanova, Mauro Mastronardi, Elisabetta Cavalcanti, Somprakas Basu, Jyoti Sharma, Tuhina Banerjee, Manisha Naithani, Navin Kumar, Sudhir Kumar Singh, Partha Pal, Rupa Banerjee, Mohan Ramchandani, Rajendra Patel, Zaheer Nabi, Swathi Kanaganti, Rajesh Gupta, Manu Tandan, Duvvuru Nageshwar Reddy

First published in London, United Kingdom, 2023 by IntechOpen
IntechOpen is the global imprint of INTECHOPEN LIMITED, registered in England and Wales, registration number: 11086078, 5 Princes Gate Court, London, SW7 2QJ, United Kingdom

British Library Cataloguing-in-Publication Data
A catalogue record for this book is available from the British Library

Additional hard and PDF copies can be obtained from orders@intechopen.com

Crohn's Disease - The Current State of the Art
Edited by Partha Pal
p. cm.
Print ISBN 978-1-83768-047-4
Online ISBN 978-1-83768-048-1
eBook (PDF) ISBN 978-1-83768-049-8

For EU product safety concerns:
IN TECH d.o.o., Prolaz Marije Krucifikse Kozulić 3, 51000 Rijeka, Croatia,
info@intechopen.com or visit our website at intechopen.com.

Meet the editor

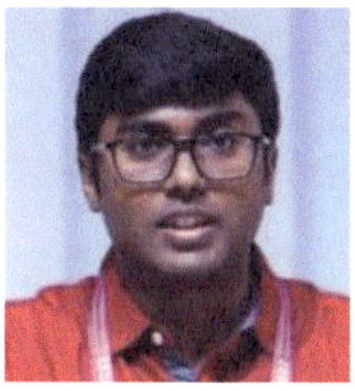

Dr. Partha Pal, MD, DNB, MRCP(UK), FASGE, is a consultant gastroenterologist and inflammatory bowel disease (IBD) specialist at the Asian Institute of Gastroenterology. His areas of interest include IBD, small bowel diseases, interventional endoscopy, and intestinal ultrasound. He has published more than 100 peer-reviewed articles on IBD, small bowel diseases, intestinal ultrasound, interventional endoscopy, and pancreatic diseases. He achieved high honors at the undergraduate and postgraduate levels, receiving awards as the best student. He won the National Young Scholar Award in 2017. Dr. Pal also received the 2021 Endoscopic Training Award from the American Society of GI Endoscopy (ASGE) and an International GI Training Grant from the American College of Gastroenterology (ACG) in 2023 for his training on interventional IBD and small bowel endoscopy.

Contents

Preface

Crohn's disease (CD) is a subgroup of inflammatory bowel disease that can affect any part of the intestine from mouth to anus. CD can be differentiated from its counterpart ulcerative colitis (UC) by transmural nature and discontinuous involvement of any part of the bowel. The sequence of events in untreated CD is chronic inflammation, stricture, fistula, and abscess formation. Early diagnosis and timely treatment can prevent the complications of this chronic, lifelong illness. This book presents a comprehensive overview of CD.

From its first description in 1913 as "chronic interstitial enteritis," the understanding of CD has evolved over the last century. Chapter 1 discusses the evolution in clinical observations, diagnosis, and treatment of CD over time.

The series of pathogenetic events leading to the development of CD as opposed to UC is not clearly known. Genetic predisposition, impaired gut permeability, and environmental factors triggering dysregulated immune response have been implicated. Rapid industrialization and improved sanitary conditions, as well as Westernization of diet and changing lifestyle factors, have been postulated to be contributing factors to rising incidence in developing countries. There is increasing evidence that these factors contribute to the development of CD by change in the gut microbiome. Chapter 2 discusses the crosstalk between dysbiosis and CD. Although there is conclusive evidence to support the bidirectional relation between gut microbiome and CD, fecal microbiota transfer has not been as successful as it has been in UC. A better understanding of the underlying factors needs evaluation.

One of the major causes of diagnostic delay in CD is the inability to differentiate it from mimics like intestinal tuberculosis (ITB) and Behcet's disease. The inability to differentiate ITB from CD, especially in tuberculosis-endemic countries, leads to treatment with empirical anti-tubercular drugs and delayed diagnosis ultimately resulting in stricture complications and high risk of surgery. Chapter 3 discusses all the differential diagnoses of CD and how to differentiate them from CD. This chapter provides valuable information for treating practitioners on early diagnosis and improving outcomes.

Once CD is suspected or initially diagnosed, mapping out the disease extent is of prime importance to guide therapy. Isolated small bowel involvement can occur in 10% of CD cases, and one-third of patients with ileocolonic disease will have small bowel involvement. Capsule endoscopy is a non-invasive, radiation-free modality with high accuracy that allows pan-enteric evaluation. Chapter 4 discusses the use of capsule endoscopy in CD.

The most dreaded phenotype of CD is the fistulizing type, which leads to fistula and abscess. The treatment options include anti-tumor necrosis factor agents along with drainage of the abscess or dilation of stricture. In recent years, endoscopic therapy for CD-related fistula and abscesses has been described. Chapter 5 summarizes the current endoscopic treatment options for CD-related fistula and abscesses.

This book presents the current state of the art of pathogenesis, diagnosis, and treatment of specific aspects of CD.

Partha Pal
Department of Medical Gastroenterology,
Asian Institute of Gastroenterology,
Hyderabad, Telangana, India

Chapter 1

Introductory Chapter: Crohn's Disease – The Current State of the Art

Partha Pal

1. Introduction

Crohn's disease (CD) is a form of inflammatory bowel disease (IBD) which is differentiated from Ulcerative colitis (UC) by its patchy and full thickness inflammation which can affect anywhere from mouth to anus. The diagnosis can be challenging in CD compared to UC due to isolated involvement of deep small bowel along with various infectious and non-infectious mimics leading to diagnostic dilemma. The current diagnostic modalities have evolved from fiberoptic endoscopy to capsule endoscopy, motorized spiral enteroscopy and even artificial intelligence assisted diagnosis from endoscopic/intestinal ultrasound images. Left untreated, it can lead to mechanical complications such as strictures and fistulas which need surgical therapy or interventional endoscopic therapies. Unlike the other counterpart (UC), CD is notorious to cause post-operative recurrence of the disease in a vast majority of the patients over time if appropriate prophylactic therapies are not initiated.

2. History of Crohn's disease

The first series of "Chronic interstitial enteritis", currently known as Crohn's disease (CD) was first reported by Scottish surgeon named Thomas Kennedy Dalziel in British Medical Journal in 1913 [1]. Nearly 20 years later in 1932, Burrill B. Crohn, Leon Ginzburg and Gordon D. Oppenheimer published the description of 14 cases of "regional enteritis" in Journal of American Medical Association [2]. According to Ginsberg, he and Oppenheimer collected 12 cases and wrote most of the manuscript and were put in touch with Crohn by the pathologist Paul Klemperer to increase the number of cases. Crohn was given the manuscript and they did not hear from him again until its was published with Crohn's name as the lead. That is how the eponym of CD was ascribed to Crohn [3]. In the next 20 years, it was recognized that CD can involve any part of the bowel apart from classical description in the ileum [3]. Since then several therapeutic and technological advances have taken place in the diagnosis and management of CD.

3. The rising burden of the disease

IBD is emerging in the developing countries where sporadic cases are reported whereas in newly industrialized countries, there is acceleration in incidence but

IntechOpen

prevalence is still low. Western countries are in stage of compounding prevalence where incidence is stable but prevalence is increasing. This is due to chronic, life-long nature of disease with low mortality. The Western countries may soon enter a stage of prevalence equilibrium in which there is balance between aging population and IBD incidence [4]. Industrialization, changing lifestyle and westernization are implicated in the rapid rise in newly industrialized countries. This gives us the opportunity to investigate the cause of the rising incidence. Epidemiological trends suggest that the rising burden of CD follows that of UC in areas where IBD is emerging [4].

4. Gut microbiome in Crohn's disease

Reduction in gut microbial diversity have been implicated in pathogenesis of CD and hence intestinal microbiota manipulation strategies have been studied as a treatment option.

Fecal microbiota transplant has not been shown to be effective in CD unlike UC. Dietary manipulation have been extensively studied although the certainty of the evidence remains low. There is emerging data on the role of partial enteral nutrition in induction and prevention of relapse in CD similar to exclusive enteral nutrition. Mediterranean diet is similar to specific carbohydrate diet although the certainty of evidence remains low [5]. A better understanding of host and microbiota interaction is warranted [6]. Currently these therapies can be used as an adjunctive therapy rather than standalone management of CD.

5. Evolution of small bowel endoscopic imaging in CD

Isolated small bowel involvement can be seen in a third of patients with CD. Although terminal ileum is involved in the majority, isolated proximal small bowel involvement is not uncommon. Small bowel evaluation have evolved from video capsule endoscopy (VCE) and balloon assisted enteroscopy to currently the motorized spiral enteroscopy. Several technological modifications of VCE have been improved the technology including patency capsule, double head capsule, three-dimensional reconstruction, sampling system, panoramic view (344 and 360 degree lateral) capsule, pan-enteric capsule, use of softwares and artificial intelligence (to reduce capsule reading time).

6. Pregnancy, fertility, sexuality and interdisciplinary management of perianal fistula

CD has been associated with higher risk of preterm delivery, small for gestational age, low birth weight and stillbirth but no increased risk of congenital abnormalities [7]. Control of disease activity is of prime importance to achieve optimal maternal and neonatal outcomes. Fertility can be decreased by disease activity, medications (male) and pelvic surgery (female). Same factors including extra-intestinal manifestations of disease can influence sexuality [8].

The management of perianal CD need multidisciplinary approach with IBD specialist, surgeon, radiologist and recently stem cell based therapies.

7. Evolution of Crohn's disease

Over the last century, IBD including CD has evolved from clinical observations to a network of advance therapies and quality of care (**Figure 1**). From the disease classification, we have moved from disease phenotypes towards genetics, immunologic typing and recently environmental typing based on microbiome. The treatments have evolved from empirical therapies to evidence based therapies, disease modifying agents and treat to target strategy to alter the natural history of the disease. Lastly we have moved from organizational funding research to collaborative efforts to understand the global phenomenon of this emerging disease. In this book, we shall focus on the various aspects of the latest development in Crohn's disease specially diagnosis, gut microbiome, small bowel capsule endoscopy and managing pregnancy.

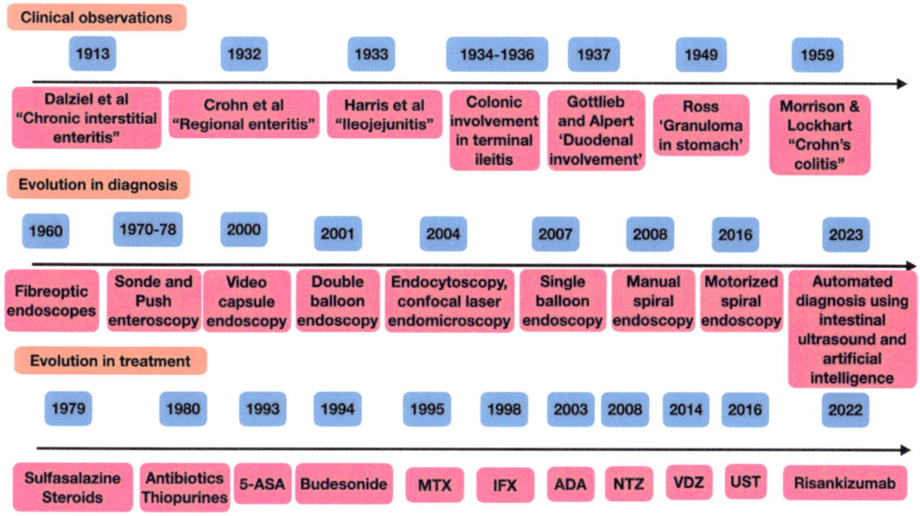

Figure 1.
Evolution of Crohn's disease from clinical observations to diverse diagnostic modalities and a network of advanced therapies. ASA-amino salicylic acid, ADA-adalimumab, IFX-infliximab, NTZ-natalizumab, VDZ-vedolizumab, UST-ustekinumab.

Author details

Partha Pal
Department of Medical Gastroenterology, Asian Institute of Gastroenterology, Hyderabad, Telangana, India

*Address all correspondence to: partha0123456789@gmail.com

References

[1] Dalziel TK. Thomas Kennedy Dalziel 1861-1924. Chronic interstitial enteritis. Diseases of the Colon & Rectum. 1989;**32**(12):1076-1078

[2] Crohn BB, Ginzburg L, Oppenheimer GD. Landmark article Oct 15, 1932. Regional ileitis. A pathological and clinical entity. Journal of the American Medical Association. 1984;**251**(1):73-79

[3] Mulder DJ, Noble AJ, Justinich CJ, Duffin JM. A tale of two diseases: The history of inflammatory bowel disease. Journal of Crohn's & Colitis. 2014;**8**(5):341-348

[4] Kaplan GG, Windsor JW. The four epidemiological stages in the global evolution of inflammatory bowel disease. Nature Reviews. Gastroenterology & Hepatology. 2021;**18**(1):56-66

[5] Limketkai BN, Godoy-Brewer G, Parian AM, et al. Dietary interventions for the treatment of inflammatory bowel diseases: An updated systematic review and meta-analysis. Clinical Gastroenterology and Hepatology. 2022

[6] Khanna S, Raffals LE. The microbiome in Crohn's disease: Role in pathogenesis and role of microbiome replacement therapies. Gastroenterology Clinics of North America. 2017;**46**(3):481-492

[7] Gaidos JKJ, Kane SV. Sexuality, fertility, and pregnancy in Crohn's disease. Gastroenterology Clinics of North America. 2017;**46**(3):531-546

[8] Lightner AL, Faubion WA, Fletcher JG. Interdisciplinary Management of Perianal Crohn's disease. Gastroenterology Clinics of North America. 2017;**46**(3):547-562

Chapter 2

Gut Microbiome and Crohn's Disease: An Enigmatic Crosstalk

Jyoti Sharma, Tuhina Banerjee, Manisha Naithani, Navin Kumar, Sudhir Kumar Singh and Somprakas Basu

Abstract

Crohn's disease (CD) is a chronic, recurrent, immune-mediated inflammatory bowel disease that demonstrates a spectrum of intestinal and extra-intestinal manifestations. The pathogenesis of CD is multifactorial and involves a complex interplay between environmental and microbiological factors in a genetically susceptible host. There is robust evidence suggesting the role of gut microbial dysbiosis in the development as well as exacerbation of CD by immune dysregulation and alteration in the immune microbiota crosstalk. Patients with CD show reduced commensal microbial diversity, along with increased numbers of pathogenic *Enterobacteriaceae* and *Proteobacteriaceae*. *Faecalibacterium prausnitzii*, an anti-inflammatory molecule-producing bacteria, is also seen in reduced numbers in patients with CD and is associated with an increased risk of recurrence. There has been a paradigm shift in the management of patients of CD, from controlling symptoms to controlling inflammation and promoting mucosal healing. Current treatment strategies aim to replace, remove, reset, or redesign the gut microbiota for the therapeutic benefits of patients with CD. These include microbial restoration therapies such as dietary modification, the use of pre-, pro-, and postbiotics, and fecal microbiota transfer (FMT). This chapter focuses on the role of gut microbiota in the pathophysiology of CD and the emerging concepts in microbial therapeutics.

Keywords: microbiome, dysbiosis, gut-immune crosstalk, microbial therapeutics, Crohn's disease

1. Introduction

Crohn's disease (CD) is a chronic relapsing inflammatory disease that can involve any part of the gut from the mouth to the anus [1]. The first documented case of CD dates back to 1761, described by Morgagni [2]. However, it was in 1932, that Crohn et al. elucidated the disease in detail [3]. There has been a rising trend in the incidence of this disease, with more than 6.8 million people affected worldwide [4]. Traditionally, known as the disease of the West, the incidence of CD has also increased in Asian and Southeast Asian countries in the past decade, owing to rapid industrialization and urbanization. The CD is primarily a disease of the young, with a second smaller peak seen in the sixth decade. A female preponderance is seen in

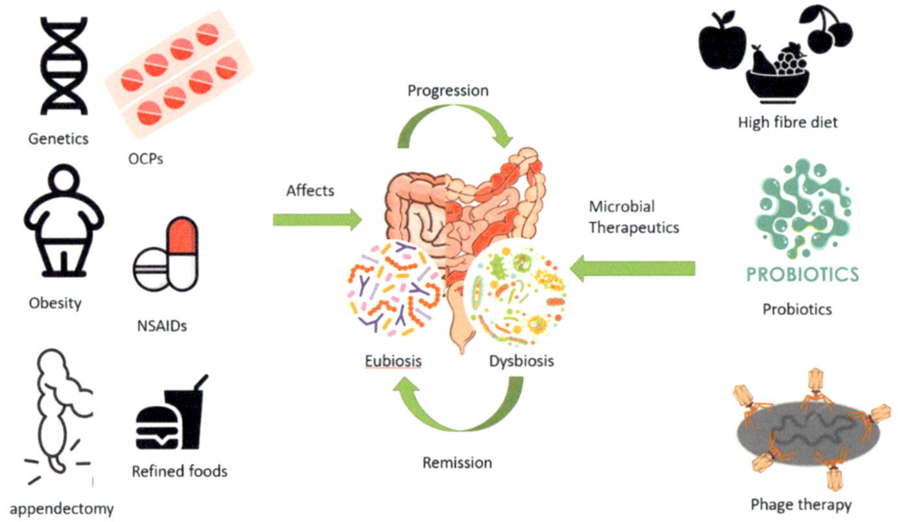

Figure 1.
Interplay of genetic, environmental factors, and microbial dysbiosis in the pathogenesis of CD and the role of microbial therapeutics and diet in the management and remission of CD.

Europe and USA, while the reverse is true in Asia. Younger females are at a lower risk of developing CD as compared to older females [5]. The exact cause of CD is still uncertain. However, the proposed pathophysiology involves an intricate relationship between the genetic, environmental, microbial, and immunological factors [6]. Recent evidence suggesting the role of gut microbial dysbiosis as an important initiator and propagator of CD has found great interest among the researchers (**Figure 1**).

Patients with CD may present with intestinal or extra-intestinal symptoms. Cardinal symptoms include crampy abdominal pain, persistent intermittent diarrhea, bleeding per rectum, weight loss, and fatigue. Severe disease is associated with intestinal strictures, fistulas, intraabdominal-abscesses, or perianal disease in the form of fistula, abscess, etc. These occur due to the transmural intestinal inflammation. Extra-intestinal involvement includes arthropathy, eye and skin manifestations, hepatobiliary and pulmonary involvement, and secondary amyloidosis [6]. The chronic relapsing and remitting course of the disease results in significant morbidity and a decreased quality of life (QOL). Individualized treatment focused on mucosal healing and aimed at remission should be undertaken, thereby improving the patient's QOL and achieving better clinical outcomes. This chapter outlines the pathophysiology, risk factors and the role of gut microbiota in the causation and progression of CD, and the recent advances in the therapeutic strategies of its management.

2. Factors promoting the development of CD

2.1 Host genetics

The onset and progression of CD are influenced by epigenetic changes in a genetically susceptible host. There is evidence suggesting a strong inheritable component of CD which has been obtained through Genome Wide Association Studies (GWAS). A total of 41 chromosomal loci involved in the maintenance of intestinal barrier, epithelial restitution, regulation of innate and adaptive immunity, autophagy, reactive oxygen species (ROS) production, microbial defense, and cellular hemostasis have been identified [7, 8]. The most extensively studied gene in the pathogenesis of CD is the *nucleotide binding oligomerization domain containing* 2 (NOD2) gene. It is responsible for immunomodulation, and its mutation is associated with the development of CD. Similarly, mutation in autophagy gene autophagy-related 16-like 1 (ATG16L1) is also associated with the development of CD, while *IL23R* gene polymorphisms increases the risk of developing CD. Early onset IBD, as seen mostly in the pediatric patients, is associated with mutations in X-linked inhibitor of apoptosis (XIAP) and interleukin 10 receptor (IL10R) genes. The prevalence of CD in certain specific population groups explains the role of genetic susceptibility to the disease. While variance in NOD-2, ATG16L1, and IL23R predominates in the western population, TNF superfamily member 15 (TNFSF15) mutation is selectively associated with CD in the Asians. Almost half of these genetic alterations are associated with diseases such as psoriasis and ankylosing spondylitis often present as extraintestinal manifestations of CD. However, this genetic variance is seen only in 10–25% of the total cases of CD which suggests the role of epigenetic factors in the causation of CD [9].

2.2 Environmental factors

The epidemiologic distribution of CD suggests a possible role of epigenetics along with genetic susceptibility of the individual. With the advent of industrialization, there has been an exponential increase in the incidence of CD, especially in the Asian and Southeast Asian countries, confirming the role of environmental factors [2]. Smoking has been extensively studied as a risk factor in CD and is associated with alterations in autophagy, gut flora, and direct toxicity to the immune and mucus-producing cells [10]. Processed foods are rich in saturated fatty acids but low in fiber, which result in intestinal mucosal inflammation and alteration in the gut microbiota. A diet rich in processed food is associated with an increased risk of CD [11]. High-fiber diet is protective in the development of CD as it is converted into short chain fatty acids (SCFA) that possess anti-inflammatory properties [9, 12]. Sedentary lifestyle and obesity are other risk factors associated with an increased risk of CD [9]. Extensive use of antibiotics in pediatric age group may alter the developing gut

Factors	Paper /year/type of study	Sample size/ no. of studies	Pd of intervention	Role
Smoking	Mahid et al. [15] (2006) Meta-analysis To et al. [10] (2015) Meta-analysis	9	Jan 1980–Jan 2006 1990–July 2015	Twofold increase in CD Early onset CD Higher postoperative disease recurrence
Low fiber diet	Lambert et al. [12] (2021) Meta-analysis	19	Jan 2000–Sept 2020	Higher risk of CD Risk reduction is greatest for fiber derived from fruits
High dietary fat/protein	Ajabnoor et al. [16] (2020) Meta-analysis	13	—	High omega-3 may reduce IBD risk (low quality evidence)

Factors	Paper /year/type of study	Sample size/ no. of studies	Pd of intervention	Role
Lifestyle	Jain et al. [17] (2019) Cohort study Nguyen et al. [18] (2019) Cohort study (nationwide)	4748 patients 42,285 patients	Since 2011 with at least 6-months follow-up Admissions between January to June 2013 and re-admissions until December 2013	Obesity is independently associated with an increased risk of persistent disease activity and relapse Obese patients with IBD had longer hospital stays
Appendectomy	Kaplan et al. [19] (2008) Meta-analysis Fantodji et al. [20] (2022) Cohort study	21 studies 400,520 patients	1966–2007 1970–1974 and followed till 2014	Still debatable
Antibiotics at early age	Ungaro et al. [13] (2014) Meta-analysis	11 studies (7208 participants)	2004–2012	Positive association if used in first year of life
Oral contraceptive use	Ortizo et al. [21] (2017) Meta-analysis	20 studies	1984–2010	Positive association
NSAID use	Moninuola et al. [22] (2018) Meta-analysis	13 studies	1974–March 2017	Positive association
Vitamin D	Pinto et al. [23] (2015) Meta-analysis Li et al. [24] (2019) Meta-analysis	14 studies (1891 participants) 55 studies	Inception—Dec 2014 1982–April 2019	Lower vitamin D levels were associated with high CD risk

Table 1.
Environmental factors and their role in the development of CD.

microbiota and may predispose to CD [13]. "Hygiene hypothesis" or exposure to a "too clean" environment during childhood causes alteration in the evolution of gut microbiota and predisposes the children to CD [14]. Indirect evidence suggesting that most of the environmental factors are associated with an alteration in the gut microbiota reaffirms their possible role in the pathogenesis of CD. However, the role of gut microbiota in either initiation or progression of CD is still uncertain (**Table 1**).

3. Pathophysiology

The pathogenesis of CD is characterized by an impaired intestinal barrier function, dysregulation of the innate and adaptive immune response, and gut microbial dysbiosis [5]. There exists a functional equilibrium between the intestinal epithelium and the luminal contents. This equilibrium is maintained by the intestinal barrier which is composed of the intestinal epithelial cells (IEC), innate immune cells, mucus layer, and the commensal gut microbiota. It is a dynamic structure that not only acts as a physical barrier but also acts as a chemical and immunological barrier against the pathogenic microbes and helps in maintaining the gut homeostasis [25].

The IECs are divided according to their functions into Goblet cells, entero-absorptive cells, Paneth cells, neuroendocrine cells, and M cells. The Goblet cells produce mucus that acts as a physical barrier and also helps in epithelial cell repair. Paneth cells are associated with maintenance of intestinal stem cell niche and secretion of antimicrobial effectors which are responsible for gut microbial homeostasis [25]. The mucosal innate immune system consists of macrophages, dendritic cells, lymphocytes, and neutrophils that form the first line of defense along with IECs. In a healthy state, the intestinal macrophages exhibit "self-tolerance" where they show attenuated response to the host microbial ligands and cytokines while retaining the bactericidal activity against pathogens. These are a special subset of macrophages that lack CD14. These promote regulatory T cell (Tregs) differentiation by producing anti-inflammatory cytokines. Tregs are a specialized subset of T cells that suppress the immune system and are responsible for maintenance of self-tolerance and homeostasis. These macrophages are also responsible for attenuation of Th1 and Th17 responses. It is observed that patients with CD exhibit another macrophage population that expresses CD14 along with dendritic cell markers, thus producing abundant pro-inflammatory cytokines such as IL-6 and TNF α and resulting in intestinal mucosal inflammation. The dendritic cells form an interface between the innate and adaptive immune system and relay signals to initiate an appropriate adaptive immune response. They perform bacterial sampling by direct dendritic cell to microbe contact which is mediated by CX3CR1-dependent mechanism. Deletion of CX3CR1 results in increased translocation of gut bacteria due to decreased lamina propria macrophages [26, 27].

The microbial products that permeate the intestinal barrier are identified by the antigen-presenting cells (APCs), which initiate a cascade of pro- and anti-inflammatory signals. This activates the local and circulating lymphocytes to migrate to the area of inflammation. The leucocyte migration occurs *via* binding of integrins on the leucocyte surface to the cellular adhesion molecules (CAMs) on the endothelium. The activated endothelium itself produces chemokines to attract leucocytes to the site of inflammation. This disturbed pro- and anti-inflammatory balance with leucocyte migration results in an exaggerated T cell response (Th1 and Th17) that is seen in CD. The APCs and macrophages secrete IL12, IL18, IL23, and TGF-β which cause differentiation of Th1 and Th17 cells. The Th1 and 17 cells secrete IL-17, IFN-ϒ, and TNF-α that in turn stimulate the APCs, macrophages, fibroblasts, and endothelial cells leading to persistent activation of the T cells [28].

Tregs and Th17 cells arise from a common precursor but have opposite actions. In normal state, TGF-β promotes Treg cell differentiation in the lamina propria depending on the local cytokines and microbial signals. But in inflammatory conditions like CD, it leads to Th17 cell differentiation promoted by the presence of other cytokines and microbial signals. This mechanism is responsible for the initiation, persistence, and relapses seen in CD [29].

4. The gut microbiome and dysbiosis

4.1 The gut microbiome

The human gut is niche to a vast variety of commensal, symbiotic, and pathogenic microbial floras that play a pivotal role in various synthetic, metabolic, and immunologic functions of the human body. Due to its immense functional plasticity, it has often been referred as the "forgotten organ." It co-evolves with the human gut and shares a complex and bi-directional interaction with the host, which helps in maintaining host homeostasis [30]. Gut bacteria form the major biomass, along with archaea, viruses, and eukaryotes. *Firmicutes*, *Bacteroidetes*, *Proteobacteria*, and *Actinobacteria* are the four predominant phyla present in the human gut of which *Firmicutes* and *Bacteroidetes* are in maximum abundance, accounting for almost 90% of the total microbiota [29]. *Firmicutes* and *Bacteroidetes*, along with *Bifidobacterium*, synthesize SCFAs, mainly butyrate, which is the principal source of energy for colonic epithelia [31]. *Bifidobacterium* also synthesizes vitamins K and B, which are essential for coagulation [32]. The gut microbiota also plays a crucial role in the development of the host immune system, which, in turn, shapes the gut microbiome [33, 34]. Animal studies have shown that mice deficient in gut microbiota exhibited impaired development of innate immune system [35]. A specific bacterium *Candidatus arthromitis*, also known as segmented filamentous bacteria (SFB), promotes the maturation of mucosal immune system, which is a significant component of the intestinal barrier [36]. *Clostridium* strains IV, XIVa, and XVIII induce Treg cell differentiation and expansion *via* butyrate production [37]. Recent research has demonstrated that *F. prausnitzii*, which belongs to Clostridium cluster IV, has an anti-inflammatory action in the human gut. It produces butyrate and anti-inflammatory bioactive molecules such as shikimic and salicylic acids, inducing the production of IL10 and inhibiting the production of IL12 and interferon-ϒ [38, 39]. In addition, the gut microbiota is also involved in the defense of the host against the intestinal pathogens. The commensal bacteria compete with the pathogenic bacteria thus preventing their colonization. This mechanism is known as "colonization resistance" [40]. They either directly inhibit them by competing for nutrients or, indirectly, by producing inhibitory substances [41]. *Bacteroides thetaiotaomicron*, an abundant commensal bacterium, utilizes the carbohydrates used by *Citrobacter rodentium*, a pathogenic bacteria, and leads to its competitive exclusion [42]. *Bacillus thuringiensis* secretes a bacteriocin that directly targets the spore forming *Clostridia* and *Bacilli* [43]. The microbial products such as lipopolysaccharides and flagellin promote the secretion of IgA from B cells, production of antimicrobial peptide, and the development of Th17 cells [44, 45].

4.2 The gut microbial dysbiosis and CD

"Dysbiosis" or an imbalance in the microbial composition alters the host-microbiota-immune crosstalk and results in disruption of host homeostasis [45]. It may occur due to various environmental factors such as dietary changes, toxins, drugs, and infections [40]. There is a reduction in the beneficial commensal bacteria and a pathological bloom of pathogenic bacteria or "pathobionts," which results in altered synthetic, metabolic, and immunomodulatory functions of the host [46]. Disruption of gut homeostasis results in increased intestinal permeability and translocation of pathogenic bacteria through the intestinal barrier. This activates the gut mucosal immune system, leading to a state of low-grade chronic inflammation [47–49]. This altered host-microbiota-immune crosstalk has been linked to the pathogenesis of various metabolic, cardiovascular, neurological, and neoplastic diseases [46]. However, their association with inflammatory bowel disease (IBD) has been a subject of interest among the researchers since the past few decades.

Gut microbial dysbiosis has surfaced as a significant aspect in the pathogenesis of IBD, exhibiting a decrease in the "alpha" or the "within-sample" diversity with a simultaneous increase in the pathobionts [49]. It is significantly affected by the geographical diversity and epigenetic factors and is more pronounced in patients with CD [50]. The taxonomic shifts in CD are mostly related to dysfunctions of microbial metabolism and bacterial protein signaling. A reduced abundance of bacterial taxa within the phyla *Firmicutes* is the most consistent finding [49]. This leads to significant reduction in SCFAs, mainly butyrate, in the gut that affects the epithelial cell growth as well as Treg cell differentiation and expansion. Other SCFA-producing bacteria such as *Bifidobacterium*, *Lactobacillus*, and *Roseburia intestinalis* are remarkably reduced in patients with CD when compared with healthy individuals. It is seen that the proportions of Clostridium clusters XIVa and IV are significantly lower in CD patients [51, 52]. *F. prausnitzii* belongs to *Clostridium* Cluster IV and possesses anti-inflammatory properties. A significant reduction in its abundance is associated with a decreased resistance of the gut against inflammatory interactions. Thus, decreased abundance of *F. prausnitzii* can be correlated with disease activity and an increased risk of recurrence after surgery [38, 52]. Studies have also shown decreased abundance of *Eubacterium rectale*, *Blautia faecis*, *Roseburia inulinivorans*, *Ruminococcus torques*, and *Clostridium lavalense* along with a decrease in families of *Christensenellaceae*, *Coriobacteriaceae*, and especially *Clostridium leptum* [50, 52–54].

Patients with CD demonstrate abundance of *Proteobacteria* such as *Enterobacteriaceae* and certain species of *Bacteriodetes*. There is a relative abundance of mucosal associated bacteria, mainly *Enteroinvasive E. coli* (EIEC) and *C. rodentium* that have adhesive properties [45]. These bacteria activate the mucosal immune system by adhering to the intestinal epithelium, thereby inducing intestinal inflammation. Decreased abundance of protective bacteria such as *C. arthromitis*, *B. thetaiotaomicron*, and *Bacillus thuringenesis* leads to proliferation of these pathobionts. Certain mucolytic bacteria such as *Ruminococcus gnavas* and *R. torques* are also increased in patients with CD [55]. Increased abundance of *Desulfovibrio*, a sulfate-reducing bacteria, is associated with intestinal epithelial damage due to production of hydrogen sulfate, thereby inducing mucosal inflammation [56]. A predominance of *Clostridium difficile* and *Bacteroides vulgates* is observed in patients with relapse of CD [57]. Abundance of pathobionts such as *Bacteroides fragilis*, strains of *Clostridium hathewayi*, *Clostridium bolteae*, *Actinomycetes* spp., *Veillonella* spp., *Intestinibacter* spp. and a significant increase in *Coprococcus* spp. is also seen in patients with CD when compared to healthy gut flora [58]. Recent studies have also isolated some strains of enterohepatic *Helicobacter* species in these patients suggesting a protective role of these strains in CD [59].

4.3 Fungal dysbiosis and CD

In addition to bacterial dysbiosis, an alteration in the mycobiome (fungal community) is also seen in these patients. Studies have shown significant decrease in the *Saccharomyces cerevisiae* abundance with a significant increase in the *Candida* spp., mainly *Candida albicans* and *tropicalis* [60]. *Malassezia restricta*, a commensal skin fungus, is also found in abundance in CD patients [61].

4.4 Viral dysbiosis and CD

Recent evidence also shows the potential role of gut virome in the pathogenesis of CD [6, 62]. The abundance of *Caudovirales* bacteriophage sequences, including *Myoviridae*, *Siphoviridae*, and *Podoviridae* detected in the intestinal washes and tissue biopsies of pediatric CD patients, may be utilized as a potential biomarker of early onset CD [63]. An increased abundance of *Synechococcus* phage S CBS1 and Retroviridae family viruses is also observed in these patients [64].

Gut microbial diversity is also affected by the medical treatment protocols of CD. Repeated antibiotic exposure is associated with a significant and consistent reduction in the gut microbial biodiversity with near absence of some specific taxa such as *Acetovibrio*, *Butyricicoccus*, *Collinsella*, *Dorea*, and *Subdoligranulum* [65]. Treatment with 5-aminosalicylic acid showed a significant decrease in *E. coli* with an increase in *Enterococcus* spp., but the results have been conflicting. Anti-TNF therapy demonstrated decreased numbers of *F. prausnitzii* and *E. coli* in some studies [57]. However, the effect of these immunomodulator therapies on the gut microbiome is little known and further research is required.

Postoperative recurrence in CD was characterized by significant abundance in the bacterial counts of *E. coli*, *Bacteroides*, and *Fusobacteria* at the neoterminal ileum. A lesser percentage of *F. prausnitzii* in the resected ileal segment was associated with an early endoscopic recurrence of CD, suggesting a microbial signature that can predict the possibility of recurrence postoperatively [66].

4.5 Genetic variants in CD and their association with microbial dysbiosis

A possible association of the gut microbiome with the genetic loci of CD has long been suspected; however, the results have not been consistent. *NOD2* gene has been extensively studied in the pathogenesis of CD. It is expressed by the Paneth cells and stimulates an immune reaction on recognizing the cell wall peptidoglycan muramyl peptide of gram-positive and gram-negative bacteria. Studies have demonstrated that NOD2 variants of CD show an increased adaptive response to microbial antigens. Risk alleles at NOD2 and ATG16L1 loci were associated with significant taxonomic shifts, especially decreased *Faecalibacterium* and *Roseburia* spp. and increased *Escherichia* spp. strains [67]. Specific genes involved in adhesion, oxidative stress responses, and utilization of mucus favor colonization of *Ruminococcus gnavus* [68]. NOD-like receptor 6 (NLRP 6) has been recognized as the key regulator of a pathobiont *Akkermansia muciniphila* that promotes the development of CD [69]. These associations were associated with a high genetic risk for CD. CLEC7A is a pattern recognition receptor that recognizes glucans with β-1,3 and β-1,6 bonds from fungi. Alteration in C-type lectin domain containing 7A (CLEC7A) is associated with altered macrophage and dendritic cell function and is associated with decreased *Lactobacillus* population [70]. Caspase recruitment domain family member 9 (CARD 9) recognizes fungal motifs and is associated with fungal dysbiosis. It is associated with decreased *Lactobacillus* population and a predominance of *Ascomycota*, *Basidiomycota*, and *Zygomycota* [71]. Alteration in nucleotide-binding oligomerization domain, *Leucine*-rich repeat, and pyrin domain containing protein (NLRP) increases susceptibility to IBD by promoting intestinal inflammation and is associated with an increased abundance of *A. muciniphila* and *Prevotellaceae* family [72]. The common CD-specific genes and their role in pathogenesis of CD and effect on the immune system and intestinal microbiota have been summarized in **Table 2**. However, consistent taxonomic shifts could not be demonstrated in further studies, thus necessitating the need for larger GWAS and higher level of evidence.

It is anticipated that portraying the compositional and functional changes in the microbial diversity will help in developing novel therapeutic options for preventing relapses and inducing remission in CD.

S. no.	Genes	Role	Role in pathogenesis of CD	Effect on the immune system	Effect of genetic variants on the intestinal microbiome
1	NOD 2	Recognizes muramyl dipeptide (MDP) that stimulates autophagy and controls bacterial replication and antigen presentation Regulation of T-cell response via MDP independent pathways	Defective recognition and removal of pathogenic bacteria Defective autophagy Decreased release of defensins	Role in innate and adaptive immunomodulation	Increased *Enterobacteriaceae*, *Erysipelotrichaceae*, *Actinobacteria* group, *Firmicutes* class, and *Bacteroides* spp. Decreased *Faecalibacterium*, *Roseburia*, *Ruminococcaceae*
2	ATG16L1	Autophagy Maintenance of intracellular homeostasis	ATG16L1T300A is associated with increased risk of CD Responsible for increased Th1 and Th17 cells in the lamina propria of ileum and colon without intestinal inflammation	Mutations are associated loss of tolerance to commensal microbiota due to increased production of IgG and IgA against commensal microbiota	Decreased abundance of *Faecalibacterium*, *Roseburia* and *Bacteroidaceae* Increased numbers of *Enterobacteriaceae* such as *Escherichia coli*; Fusobacteriaceae, increase in *Lachnospiraceae*
3	IRGM	Responsible for autophagy Maintenance of intracellular homeostasis	Defective autophagy Decreased production of antimicrobial peptide Abnormal secretory granule development	Plays a role in innate immune response	Decreased abundance of *Roseburia*
4	IL23R [73]	Maintains T-cell dependent immunity by encoding a subunit of IL-23 that is involved in Th-17 cell generation	Role in autoimmunity by expansion of proinflammatory Th17 cells in CD	Responsible for persistent production of pro-inflammatory mediators like *IL6*, *IL12*, *IL17*, *INF-γ*, *TNF-α* and *IL23*	Decreased abundance of *Christensenellaceae*, *Bacteroides caccae* and *Oscillospira*
5	IL-10R [74, 75]	Essential for immune homeostasis in colon	Causes extensive perianal and colonic inflammation Leads to very early onset IBD (VEO-IBD) and extensive perianal disease	Role in immunomodulation, suppresses proliferation and cytokine secretion	Increased numbers of *Enterococcus faecalis*, *E. coli*, and *Helicobacter hepaticus*
6	CLEC7A	Pattern recognition receptor Recognizes various glucan bonds from fungi (β-1,3 and β-1,6 bonds)	Associated with altered macrophage and dendritic cell activity Associated with fungal dysbiosis	Role in innate immunity	Decreased abundance of nonpathogenic *Lactobacillus, Saccharomyces* Increased numbers of *Enterobacteriaceae*, *Candida*, and *Trichosporon*

S. no.	Genes	Role	Role in pathogenesis of CD	Effect on the immune system	Effect of genetic variants on the intestinal microbiome
7	CARD9	Recognizes viral, bacterial, and especially fungal motifs	Associated with fungal dysbiosis	Enhances production of IL-1β and IL-23p19 subunit	Decreased colonies of *Lactobacillus* Dominant *Ascomycota*, *Basidiomycota*, and *Zygomycota*
8	NLRP [72]	Has a molecular domain that helps in self oligomerization and has ATPase activity Can sense endogenous alarmins and microbial ligands	Promotes intestinal inflammation Increases susceptibility to colitis in murine models	Activation of IL-1 family cytokines	Key regulator of *Akkermansia muciniphila*, *Prevotellaceae* family Increased *S. thuringiensis*, *Clostridium*, *Rod bacteria*, and *Proteobacteria*
9	PTPN 2 [76]	Associated with autophagy	Defective autophagosome formation and bacterial elimination Promotes T cell differentiation into Th1 and Th17 types Associated with increased levels of IFN-γ, IL-17, and IL-22 in the serum and intestinal mucosa	High levels of *INF-γ*, *IL17* and *IL22* Role in innate and adaptive immunity	Reduced *Faecalibacterium*, *Bilophila*, *Coprococcus*, *Erysipelotrichaeceae*, *Clostridiales*, and *Ruminococcaceae* *Bacteroides* were increased in number
10	LRRK-2 [77]	Involved in endocytosis, phagocytosis, and autophagocytosis, lysosomal function Also implicated in intracellular trafficking	Activation of LRRK is associated with increased dendrtitic cell activation, increased expression and release of pro-inflammatory molecules like *IL2* and *TNF-α*	Production of IL-2 and TNF-α and activation of dendritic cells	Increased numbers of *Listeria monocytogenes* and *Salmonella Typhimurium*

Abbreviations: IRGM, immunity related GTPase-M; PTPN-2, protein tyrosine phosphate non-receptor-2; LRRK-2, leucine-rich repeat kinase-2 [70–72].

Table 2.
Genetic variants and their association with intestinal microbiota in CD.

5. Nutrition in CD

Nutrition plays an important role in the management of CD. Dietary changes can influence the gut microbiota and help in restoring the gut homeostasis [78, 79]. In addition, nutritional management is also important in view of CD-associated malnutrition, which results from decreased absorption, intestinal dysbiosis, and CD-related symptoms such as loss of appetite, nausea, and vomiting. Specific dietary strategies have been advised for the management of CD.

5.1 Diets for nutritional optimization in CD

Enteral nutrition (EN) is a liquid dietary regimen that can be given in three formulations, depending on the protein and fat content. These formulations include elemental (easily absorbable low-fat nutrients such as amino acids, mono- or oligosaccharides, and medium-chain triglycerides), semielemental (peptides of different chain length, simple sugars, glucose polymers or starch, and medium-chain triglycerides), and polymeric (whole proteins, complex carbohydrates, and long-chain triglycerides). These formulations are particularly recommended during CD relapses for 6–8 weeks to induce disease remission. These formulations are also advised as a maintenance diet during the remission phase in addition to the usual diet. This type of diet affects the gut microbiota and reduces gut bacterial dysbiosis.

Parenteral nutrition (PN) provides nutrients including macronutrients, micronutrients, and electrolytes through a venous access. Exclusive parenteral nutrition is advised during acute inflammatory phase of CD to provide bowel rest or in conditions such as partial obstruction, high-output fistulae, and bowel ischemia, where the use of enteral nutrition is contraindicated. It is also used as a supplement in patients where enteral nutrition is inadequate to fulfill the energy requirement. Thus, EN often represents the main dietary option, alone, or in association with PN.

5.2 Specific carbohydrate diet

Apart from treatment of celiac disease, this diet is also used in the management of IBD. It includes monosaccharides, dairy products with low lactose content, meat, eggs, oil, and amylose rich vegetables. Products rich in sucrose, maltose, isomaltose, and lactose, along with potatoes, corn, soy, food additives, and preservatives, must be avoided. Studies have shown that this diet improves IBD symptoms and quality of life, and help in maintaining remission.

5.3 Low fermentable, oligosaccharides, disaccharides, monosaccharides, and polyols (FODMAP) diet

This diet mainly excludes short-chain carbohydrates and limits consumption of honey, apples, watermelon, dates, lentils, and legumes. The drawback of low FODMAP diet is reduced intake of common prebiotics, such as inulin, fructo-oligosaccharides, and fructose. The low FODMAP diet is advisable in patients with quiescent IBD.

5.4 Semivegetarian diet

It is primarily a vegetarian dietary regimen which strongly limits meat and fish, without eliminating them. This diet consists of vegetables, fruits, cereals, eggs, yoghurt, and milk, and excludes processed and refined foods. It is advised as a maintenance treatment in patients with clinical remission.

5.5 Low fat/fiber limited exclusion (LOFFLEX) diet

This is a form of elemental diet which is used to find the potential trigger of CD by reintroducing specific nutrients. It can be customized accordingly by exclusion of nutrients that are commonly considered as triggers of CD, in a well-structured protocol.

Overall, the abovementioned dietary regimens play an essential role in the treatment of IBD, particularly CD. It is apparent that food components have the ability to modulate metabolic pathways, stimulate gene expression, and modify the microbiota composition. Liquid diet is the primary therapy in the management of CD as it reduces inflammation and promotes mucosal healing and helps in reducing the postoperative complications.

6. Therapeutic perspective

Ever since the understanding of natural history of CD became clearer, the therapeutic goals have shifted from controlling symptoms to controlling the inflammation and promoting mucosal healing. The treatment strategies have become more personalized and individual-based, thereby leading to better clinical outcomes. The significant role of gut microbiota in the pathogenesis of CD has influenced the development of novel therapeutic options that selectively target the gut microbiome (**Table 3**). These microbiota-targeted strategies aim at the diagnostic, prognostic, and therapeutic aspects of CD. These treatment strategies aim to replace, remove, reset, or redesign the gut microbiota for therapeutic benefits of patients with CD.

Decreased abundance	Increased abundance
Firmicutes spp.	*Escherichia coli (EHEC O157)*
Bifidobacterium	*Citrobacter rodentium*
Candidatus arthromitis	*Bacteroides fragilis*
Faecalibacterium prausnitzii	*Ruminococcus torques*
Bacteroides thetaiotamicron	*Ruminococcus gnavas*
Bacillus thuringenesis	*Desulfovibrio*
Blautia faecis	*Actinomyces*
Eubacterium rectale	*Veilonella*
Roseburia intestinalis	*Intestinibacter*
Clostridium lavalense	*Closridium hathewayi*
Christensenellaceae	*Clostridium boltae*
Coriobacteriaceae	*Coprococcus*
Clostridium leptum	*Clostridium difficile*
	Virome: *Caudovirales* *Synechococcus* phage S CBS1 Retroviridae family viruses
Mycome: *Saccharomyces cerevisiae*	Mycome: *Candida albicans* *Candida tropicalis* *Malassezia restricta*

Table 3.
Gut microbiota in Crohn's disease.

6.1 Potential biomarkers

Various noninvasive tests such as serum markers, fecal biomarkers, and radiological imaging are available for the diagnosis and monitoring the progression of CD. However, most of these serum and fecal biomarkers are limited to active disease and are surrogate markers; thus, their response to therapy is highly variable. Evaluation of specific microbial biomarkers would help in precise diagnosis and patient stratification in CD. Studies have suggested increased *Faecalibacterium nucleatum* and decreased *F. prausnitzii* counts as a valuable marker for CD [51]. Recent data analysis has identified *Gammaproteobacteria*, *Enterococcus*, and *Enterococcaceae* as potential biomarkers of IBD. Bacterial genera *Collinsella* and *Methanobrevibacter* can be used for differentiation between UC and CD [80, 81]. *F. prausnitzii* and *E. coli* can be used to differentiate between ileal and colonic CD. Ileal CD is characterized by a lower abundance of *F. prausnitzii* with a relative higher abundance of *E. coli* as compared to colonic CD. It has also been noted that AIEC is more abundantly found in the inflamed ileal mucosa of the patients suffering with CD. *Faecalibacterium* and *Papillibacter* can be used as indicators of disease status [82, 83]. They may serve as microbial signatures to diagnose and differentiate between uncertain cases of ulcerative colitis (UC), CD, and irritable bowel syndrome [84]. The microbial shifts may act as biomarkers to predict the outcome of the disease. However, due to high microbial diversity, the predictive value of these biomarkers is considerably less. Thus, they are currently not recommended as a first-line assessment for the diagnosis of CD.

6.2 Live biotherapeutic products (LBP)

Probiotics are selected viable microorganisms that modulate the intestinal microbiota and exert a beneficial effect on the host by modulating the intestinal microbiota and alleviating intestinal dysbiosis [85]. Theoretically, probiotics produce metabolites that inhibit the growth of the pathobionts and promote the growth of commensal bacteria, thus restoring the normal gut microbiome. They also induce an anti-inflammatory effect and improve and restore gut barrier function [86]. Various bacterial strains have been tested in human clinical trials, including *Bifidobacterium* spp., *E. coli* Nissle 1917, *Saccharomyces boulardii*, and *Lactobacillus* spp. and found to have beneficial effect on gut health [87]. However, their efficacy in the management of Crohn's disease has been controversial. Clinical trials have suggested a positive clinical effect of VSL#3, a probiotic containing four *Lactobacilli* (three *Bifidobacterium* spp. and *Streptococcus salivarius* subsp. thermophilus) in patients with active UC. However, it failed to prove its efficacy in patients with CD. These incongruences can in part be explained by the variety of probiotics used. It is imperative to note that the human gut-derived microbiota will have the best colonization and the most compatible therapeutic effect in patients with CD. Traditionally, the probiotics have been isolated from various dairy and nondairy products. These next-generation probiotics are derived from human feces or saliva and have a higher resistance to gastric enzymes and bile salts. In addition, they are also beneficial in patients with lactose intolerance [88, 89]. However, the feces-derived probiotics are not easily accepted by the patients due to the general perception of it being unhygienic. Recently, the concept of "synbiotics" has surfaced, which means adding a prebiotic to the probiotic [90]. A prebiotic is a substance selectively utilized by the probiotic, such as insulin and fructo-oligosaccharides [85, 86], and its use significantly improves remission rates, clinical activity, and histological scores in active CD [91]. Postbiotics are metabolites produced by live microbes and are essential in maintaining the gut homeostasis. They include organic acids such as short-chain fatty acids (SCFA), tryptophan, and some bacteriocins. They exert an anti-inflammatory and anti-oxidant effect in the human gut and inhibit the growth of pathobionts. Administration of SCFAs and tryptophan have shown remission of inflammation in animal models; however, its efficacy in humans is controversial and under trial [92].

6.3 Live bacterial consortia (gut 103 and 108)

Gut 103 and 108 are used to supplement deficient microbiota and correct dysbiosis in patients with CD. Gut 103 consists of 17 bacterial strains, while Gut 108 is a purified version of Gut 103 and utilizes 11 human bacteria associated with the 17 strains. These bacterial formulations have shown to decrease pathobionts, expand the resident flora, decrease mucosal inflammation, and re-establish gut homeostasis. Moreover, these formulations allow the bacteria to stay longer in the colon as compared to other probiotics thereby increasing their efficacy [93].

6.4 Antibiotic therapy

Antibiotic therapy has shown benefits in some patient groups with active CD. They aim at controlling the pathogenic bacterial blooms, thereby reducing the gut microbial dysbiosis. This helps in reducing the gut mucosal inflammation, thereby decreasing the disease activity and inducing remission. Anti-mycobacterial drugs, fluoroquinolones, and rifaximin have shown positive results in active CD remission in certain population groups [94]. A small randomized controlled trial compared the effect of Ciprofoxacin and Mesalazine in patients with mild to moderate CD and observed complete remission with Ciprofloxacin [95]. Another randomized trial showed early benefits of antibiotics in 213 patients receiving either Clarithromycin, Rifabutin, or Clofazimine, with no significant difference in the relapse rates were noted in follow-up [96]. Antibiotic therapy is also used to prevent postoperative recurrence of CD and in treatment of complications of CD like perianal abscess and fistula. The current limitation of antibiotic therapy is the collateral damage to the healthy gut microbiome due to its nonspecific effect and development of antibiotic resistance. Further research is required to establish a definitive role of antibiotics in the management of CD.

6.5 Phage therapy

Phage therapy consists of using highly specific lytic bacteriophages to target strains within one bacterial species. This therapy is more advantageous than antibiotic therapy as it targets a specific strain of pathogenic bacteria with a limited impact on the normal gut microbiota [97]. Enteroinvasive *E. coli* (EIEC) are abundantly present in the ileum of patients with CD and have been linked to gut mucosal inflammation. Specific bacteriophages against EIEC have been isolated, and it has been observed that administration of "phage cocktail" (2×10^9 PFU/mL) could significantly reduce EIEC colonization [98]. A recent study on transgenic mice model of dextran sulfate sodium (DSS)-induced colitis showed that a single-day treatment with oral phage cocktail significantly reduced the colonization of EIEC and reduced intestinal symptoms over a period of 2 weeks. Another crossover trial suggested that administration of phage cocktail over 28 days selectively reduced fecal EIEC without disrupting the commensal gut microbiota [99]. Federici et al. developed an orally administered lytic five-phage combination that targets the antibiotic resistant *Klebsiella pneumoniae* clade and demonstrated its feasibility in the management of IBD [100]. Although promising, the major concern of phage therapy is safety and the dosing schedule which remains as future challenges.

6.6 Bacterial vectors

The role of genetically engineered bacteria as a vector for therapeutic agents has been an area of interest. *Lactococcus lactis* is an innocuous vector as it is noninfective and noninvasive for the human body and hence has been widely studied. Oral formulations of genetically engineered *L. lactis* secreting IL-10, AG011 are undergoing various clinical trials and have been reported to reduce adverse drug reactions [101]. Other substances recombined into *L. lactis* are murine TNF neutralizing antibodies and IL-1 antagonists, which have shown promising results [102, 103].

6.7 Fecal microbiota transplantation (FMT)

FMT aims to restore the gut microbiota in CD patients by transferring these from a healthy donor to the affected recipient. The prevailing concept is that FMT might correct the gut microbial dysbiosis and lead to restoration of normal gut microbiota [104]. FMT has shown high efficacy in patients with recurrent *C. difficile* infection and has raised a possibility of its benefit in other diseases associated with gut dysbiosis like CD [105]. The inoculum can be given as fresh or frozen sample via various enteral routes. A recent systematic review published in 2021 concluded a 79% clinical response rate and a 62% clinical remission rate in CD patients. Moreover, it was noted that the rate of clinical remission was higher in patients treated with fresh stools as compared to frozen stools [48]. FMT is generally well tolerated and safe in CD with rare serious adverse effects. However, there is meager evidence on the long-term immunological effects of FMT. There are also certain limitations to this therapy such as heterogeneity in the technique, frequency of administration, and the ideal time to perform FMT. These factors affect the clinical outcome of treatment. Moreover, the multifactorial pathogenesis of CD and the dubious role of dysbiosis as a cause or consequence of the disease limit the effectiveness of this therapy. Thus, larger and well-designed studies and clinical trials are necessary to evaluate the effectiveness and optimal technique of FMT.

6.8 Role of *F. prausnitzii*

F. prausnitzii belongs to *Clostridium* cluster IV and is one of the main butyrate producers of the human gut. It exhibits anti-inflammatory properties by producing butyrate and inducing a tolerogenic cytokine profile. This includes decreased secretion of IL-12 and IFN-ϒ and increased secretion of IL-10 [38]. *F. prausnitzii* along with *E. coli* (F-E index) can help differentiate CD from irritable bowel syndrome (IBS) and UC. The F-E index can also be used to distinguish between ileal and colonic CD. *F. prausnitzii* levels can be used as a biomarker to assess disease progression and clinical response [39]. High fecal *F. prausnitzii* counts are associated with a lower CD activity. *F. prausnitzii* has shown promising results as a good microbial biomarker; however, larger well-designed studies are essential to achieve a consensus.

7. Future direction

Understanding dysbiosis and specific microbial pathways in the causation of CD has led to adaptation of more targeted treatment strategies. Microbiome-targeted therapies aim at diagnosis, treatment, stratification, and assessment of high-risk population groups.

Profiling the gut microbiota may provide essential information related to the pathogenesis and treatment efficacy in patients with CD. Microbiome multiomics provide information on the interaction of specific microbiota with its environment and may help in understanding the functional aspect of dysbiosis in CD. They help in identifying and isolating the microbiota. Various methods for isolation of the gut microbiome have emerged lately. Organoids in 2D culture and "Gut on chip" are novel techniques developed to isolate the gut microbes and monitor host-microbial interactions [58]. Microbial multiomics, combined with precision medicine provides a more specific, "personalized" treatment to an individual and predicts a better treatment response and clinical outcome.

There is ongoing research on the safety and routes of administration of FMT. Oral FMT capsules have emerged as a novel noninvasive method for FMT. A recent meta-analysis examining the safety and efficacy of oral FMT capsules concluded that this method is easy with an overall efficacy of 82.1% [106]. However, safety of FMT is a big concern, as the donor feces may contain unknown pathogenic microbiota. Due to these concerns, a Canadian group has mass cultivated probiotics from processed feces which has shown positive results in *C. difficile* colitis [106]. However, these probiotics are still under speculation and need further research to determine its safety.

8. Conclusion

There is compelling evidence demonstrating the association of gut microbial dysbiosis in the pathogenesis of CD; however, its causal relationship is still uncertain. Microbial dysbiosis has been observed in asymptomatic patients with genetic susceptibility and patients with an inactive disease, suggesting that the microbial changes are present long before inflammation. This indicates the potential role of microbial dysbiosis in the causation of CD. Moreover, postoperative recurrence at neo-terminal ileum again suggests the causal role of dysbiosis in CD. The advent of bacteriotherapy has led to more targeted treatment strategies in patients with CD. However, the biggest challenge that still exists is the inconsistency and heterogeneity of data on the dysbiotic microbial composition that limits effective microbial therapies. In addition, their role in predicting the response to therapy is still unanswered. It is anticipated that better designed studies and advanced genetic sequencing technology will lead to a more defined role of gut microbiome in the pathogenesis and treatment of CD.

Conflict of interest

The authors report no conflict of interest.

Author details

Jyoti Sharma[1], Tuhina Banerjee[2], Manisha Naithani[3], Navin Kumar[3], Sudhir Kumar Singh[3] and Somprakas Basu[3*]

1 All India Institute of Medical Sciences Delhi, Delhi, India

2 Banaras Hindu University, Varanasi, India

3 All India Institute of Medical Sciences Rishikesh, India

*Address all correspondence to: somprakas.surg@aiimsrishikesh.edu.in

IntechOpen

References

[1] Fichera A, Krane MK, editors. Crohn's disease: Basic principles. 1st ed. Switzerland: Springer; 2015. p. 306. DOI: 10.1007/978-3-319-14181-7

[2] Jairath V, Feagan BG. Global burden of inflammatory bowel disease. The Lancet Gastroenterology & Hepatology [Internet]. 2020;**5**(1):2-3. DOI: 10.1016/S2468-1253(19)30358-9

[3] Park SH. Update on the epidemiology of inflammatory bowel disease in Asia: Where are we now? Intestinal Research. 2022;**20**(2):159-164

[4] Molodecky NA, Soon IS, Rabi DM, Ghali WA, Ferris M, Chernoff G, et al. Increasing incidence and prevalence of the inflammatory bowel diseases with time, based on systematic review. Gastroenterology [Internet]. 2012;**142**(1):46-54.e42. DOI: 10.1053/j.gastro.2011.10.001

[5] Greuter T, Manser C, Pittet V, Vavricka SR, Biedermann L. Gender differences in inflammatory bowel disease. Digestion. 2020;**101**(Suppl. 1):98-104

[6] Roda G, Chien Ng S, Kotze PG, et al. Crohn's disease. Nature Reviews Disease Primers [Internet]. April 2020;**6**(1):26. DOI: 10.1038/s41572-020-0156-2

[7] Liu JZ, Van Sommeren S, Huang H, Ng SC, Alberts R, Takahashi A, et al. Association analyses identify 38 susceptibility loci for inflammatory bowel disease and highlight shared genetic risk across populations. Nature Genetics. 2015;**47**(9):979-986

[8] Huang H, Fang M, Jostins L, Umićević Mirkov M, Boucher G, Anderson CA, et al. Fine-mapping inflammatory bowel disease loci to single-variant resolution. Nature [Internet]. 2017;**547**(7662):173-178. DOI: 10.1038/nature22969

[9] Gajendran M, Loganathan P, Catinella AP, Hashash JG. A comprehensive review and update on Crohn's disease. Disease-a-Month [Internet]. 2018;**64**(2):20-57. DOI: 10.1016/j.disamonth.2017.07.001

[10] To N, Gracie DJ, Ford AC. Systematic review with meta-analysis: The adverse effects of tobacco smoking on the natural history of Crohn's disease. Alimentary Pharmacology & Therapeutics. 2016;**43**(5):549-561

[11] Tomasello G, Mazzola M, Leone A, Sinagra E, Zummo G, Farina F, et al. Nutrition, oxidative stress and intestinal dysbiosis: Influence of diet on gut microbiota in inflammatory bowel diseases. Biomedical Papers. 2016;**160**(4):461-466

[12] Lambert K, Pappas D, Miglioretto C, Javadpour A, Reveley H, Frank L, et al. Systematic review with meta-analysis: Dietary intake in adults with inflammatory bowel disease. Alimentary Pharmacology & Therapeutics. 2021;**54**(6):742-754

[13] Ungaro R, Bernstein CN, Gearry R, Hviid A, Kolho KL, Kronman MP, et al. Antibiotics associated with increased risk of new-onset Crohn's disease but not ulcerative colitis: A meta-analysis. The American Journal of Gastroenterology. 2014;**109**(11):1728-1738

[14] Cholapranee A, Ananthakrishnan AN. Environmental hygiene and risk of inflammatory bowel diseases.

Inflammatory Bowel Diseases. 2016;**22**(9):2191-2199

[15] Mahid SS, Minor KS, Soto RE, Hornung CA, Galandiuk S. Smoking and inflammatory bowel disease: A meta-analysis. Mayo Clinic Proceedings. 2006;**81**(11):1462-1471

[16] Ajabnoor SM, Thorpe G, Abdelhamid A, Hooper L. Long-term effects of increasing omega-3, omega-6 and total polyunsaturated fats on inflammatory bowel disease and markers of inflammation: A systematic review and meta-analysis of randomized controlled trials. European Journal of Nutrition [Internet]. 2021;**60**(5):2293-2316. DOI: 10.1007/s00394-020-02413-y

[17] Jain A, Nguyen NH, Proudfoot JA, et al. Impact of Obesity on Disease Activity and Patient-Reported Outcomes Measurement Information System (PROMIS) in Inflammatory Bowel Diseases. American Journal of Gastroenterol. 2019;**114**(4):630-639

[18] Nguyen NH, Ohno-Machado L, Sandborn WJ, Singh S. Obesity is independently associated with higher annual burden and costs of hospitalization in patients with inflammatory bowel diseases. Clinical Gastroenterology and Hepatology [Internet]. 2019;**17**(4):709-718.e7. DOI: 10.1016/j.cgh.2018.07.004

[19] Kaplan GG, Jackson T, Sands BE, Frisch M, Andersson RE, Korzenik J. The risk of developing Crohn's disease after an appendectomy: A meta-analysis. The American Journal of Gastroenterology. 2008;**103**(11):2925-2931

[20] Fantodji C, Jantchou P, Parent ME, Rousseau MC. Appendectomy and risk for inflammatory bowel disease: Effect of age and time post appendectomy—A cohort study. BMJ Open Gastroenterology. 2022;**9**(1):1-8

[21] Ortizo R, Lee SY, Nguyen ET, Jamal MM, Bechtold MM, Nguyen DL. Exposure to oral contraceptives increases the risk for development of inflammatory bowel disease: A meta-analysis of case-controlled and cohort studies. European Journal of Gastroenterology & Hepatology. 2017;**29**(9):1064-1070

[22] Moninuola OO, Milligan W, Lochhead P, Khalili H. Systematic review with meta-analysis: Association between acetaminophen and nonsteroidal anti-inflammatory drugs (NSAIDs) and risk of Crohn's disease and ulcerative colitis exacerbation. Alimentary Pharmacology & Therapeutics. 2018;**47**(11):1428-1439

[23] Del Pinto R, Pietropaoli D, Chandar AK, Ferri C, Cominelli F. Association between inflammatory bowel disease and vitamin D deficiency. Inflammatory Bowel Diseases. 2015;**21**(11):2708-2717

[24] Li XX, Liu Y, Luo J, Huang ZD, Zhang C, Fu Y. Vitamin D deficiency associated with Crohn's disease and ulcerative colitis: A meta-analysis of 55 observational studies. Journal of Translational Medicine. 2019;**17**(1):1-19

[25] Vancamelbeke M, Vermeire S. The intestinal barrier: A fundamental role in health and disease. Expert Review of Gastroenterology & Hepatology. 2017;**11**(9):821-834

[26] Peterson LW, Artis D. Intestinal epithelial cells: Regulators of barrier function and immune homeostasis. Nature Reviews Immunology [Internet]. 2014;**14**(3):141-153. DOI: 10.1038/nri3608

[27] Jakobsson HE, Rodríguez-Piñeiro AM, Schütte A, Ermund A, Boysen P, Bemark M, et al. The composition of the gut microbiota shapes the colon mucus barrier. EMBO Reports. 2015;**16**(2):164-177

[28] DeFilippis EM, Longman R, Harbus M, Dannenberg K, Scherl EJ. Crohn's disease: Evolution, epigenetics, and the emerging role of microbiome-targeted therapies. Current Gastroenterology Reports. 2016;**18**(3):1-9

[29] de Souza Heitor SP, Claudio F. Immunopathogenesis of IBD: Current state of the art. Nature Reviews. Gastroenterology & Hepatology. 2017;**14**(1):3

[30] Jandhyala SM, Talukdar R, Subramanyam C, Vuyyuru H, Sasikala M, Reddy DN. Role of the normal gut microbiota. World Journal of Gastroenterology. 2015;**21**(29):8836-8847

[31] Silva JPB, Navegantes-Lima KC, Oliveira ALB, Rodrigues DVS, Gaspar SLF, Monteiro VVS, et al. Protective mechanisms of butyrate on inflammatory bowel disease. Current Pharmaceutical Design. 2018;**24**(35):4154-4166

[32] Ramakrishna BS. Role of the gut microbiota in human nutrition and metabolism. Journal of Gastroenterology and Hepatology. 2013;**28**(S4):9-17

[33] Wu HJ, Wu E. The role of gut microbiota in immune homeostasis and autoimmunity. Gut Microbes. 2012;**3**(1):4-14

[34] Honda K, Littman DR. The microbiota in adaptive immune homeostasis and disease. Nature. 2016;**535**(7610):75-84

[35] Fomby P, Cherlin AJ. Role of microbiota in immunity and inflammation. National Institutes of Health. 2011;**72**(2):181-204

[36] Ivanov II, Atarashi K, Manel N, Brodie EL, Shima T, Karaoz U, et al. Induction of intestinal Th17 cells by segmented filamentous bacteria. Cell [Internet]. 2009;**139**(3):485-498. DOI: 10.1016/j.cell.2009.09.033

[37] Atarashi K, Tanoue T, Oshima K, Suda W, Nagano Y, Nishikawa H, et al. Treg induction by a rationally selected mixture of Clostridia strains from the human microbiota. Nature. 2013;**500**(7461):232-236

[38] Sokol H, Pigneur B, Watterlot L, Lakhdari O, Bermúdez-Humarán LG, Gratadoux JJ, et al. Faecalibacterium prausnitzii is an anti-inflammatory commensal bacterium identified by gut microbiota analysis of Crohn disease patients. Proceedings of the National Academy of Sciences of the United States of America. 2008;**105**(43):16731-16736

[39] Parsaei M, Sarafraz N, Moaddab SY, Ebrahimzadeh LH. The importance of Faecalibacterium prausnitzii in human health and diseases. New Microbes and New Infections [Internet]. 2021;**43**:100928. DOI: 10.1016/j.nmni.2021.100928

[40] Pickard JM, Zeng MY, Caruso R, Núñez G. Gut microbiota: Role in pathogen colonization, immune responses, and inflammatory disease. Immunological Reviews. 2017;**279**(1):70-89

[41] Buffie CG, Pamer EG. Microbiota-mediated colonization resistance against intestinal pathogens. Nature Reviews Immunology [Internet]. 2013;**13**(11):790-801. DOI: 10.1038/nri3535

[42] Kamada N, Kim YG, Sham HP, Vallance BA, Puente JL, Martens EC, et al. Regulated virulence controls the ability of a pathogen to compete with the gut microbiota. Science (80–). 2012;**336**(6086):1325-1329

[43] Huang T, Zhang X, Pan J, Su X, Jin X, Guan X. Purification and characterization of a novel cold shock protein-like bacteriocin synthesized

by Bacillus thuringiensis. Scientific Reports [Internet]. 2016;**6**(April):1-14. DOI: 10.1038/srep35560

[44] Pilmis B, Le Monnier A, Zahar JR. Gut microbiota, antibiotic therapy and antimicrobial resistance: A narrative review. Microorganisms. 2020;**8**(2):1-17

[45] Melissa K, Carles U, Al E. Bacterial flagellin stimulates TLR5-dependent defense against vancomycin-resistant enterococcus infection. Bone. 2006;**23**(1):1-7

[46] Sharma J, Huda F, Naithani M, Singh SK, Kumar N, Basu S. Role of gut microbiome and enteric bacteria in gallbladder cancer. In: Rodrigo L, editor. Immunology of the GI Tract—Recent Advances [Internet]. London: IntechOpen; 2022. Available from: https://www.intechopen.com/chapters/81344. DOI: 10.5772/intechopen.104404

[47] Llewellyn SR, Britton GJ, Contijoch EJ, Vennaro OH, Mortha A, Colombel JF, et al. Interactions between diet and the intestinal microbiota alter intestinal permeability and colitis severity in mice. Gastroenterology [Internet]. 2018;**154**(4):1037-1046.e2. DOI: 10.1053/j.gastro.2017.11.030

[48] Cheng F, Huang Z, Wei W, Li Z. Fecal microbiota transplantation for Crohn's disease: a systematic review and meta-analysis. Techniques in Coloproctology. 2021;**25**:495-504

[49] Kostic AD, Xavier RJ, Gevers D. The microbiome in inflammatory bowel disease: Current status and the future ahead. Gastroenterology [Internet]. 2014;**146**(6):1489-1499. DOI: 10.1053/j.gastro.2014.02.009

[50] Qiu P, Ishimoto T, Fu L, Zhang J, Zhang Z, Liu Y. The gut microbiota in inflammatory bowel disease. Frontiers in Cellular and Infection Microbiology. 2022;**12**(February):1-14

[51] Takahashi K, Nishida A, Fujimoto T, Fujii M, Shioya M, Imaeda H, et al. Reduced abundance of butyrate-producing bacteria species in the fecal microbial community in Crohn's disease. Digestion. 2016;**93**(1):59-65

[52] Varela E, Manichanh C, Gallart M, Torrejón A, Borruel N, Casellas F, et al. Colonisation by Faecalibacterium prausnitzii and maintenance of clinical remission in patients with ulcerative colitis. Alimentary Pharmacology & Therapeutics. 2013;**38**(2):151-161

[53] Pittayanon R, Lau JT, Leontiadis GI, Tse F, Yuan Y, Surette M, et al. Differences in gut microbiota in patients with vs without inflammatory bowel diseases: A systematic review. Gastroenterology [Internet]. 2020;**158**(4):930-946.e1. DOI: 10.1053/j.gastro.2019.11.294

[54] Rolhion N, Darfeuille-Michaud A. Adherent-invasive Escherichia coli in inflammatory bowel disease. Inflammatory Bowel Diseases. 2007;**13**(10):1277-1283

[55] Liu S, Zhao W, Lan P, Mou X. The microbiome in inflammatory bowel diseases: From pathogenesis to therapy. Protein & Cell [Internet]. 2021;**12**(5):331-345. DOI: 10.1007/s13238-020-00745-3

[56] Loubinoux J, Bronowicki JP, Pereira IAC, Mougenel JL, Le Faou AE. Sulfate-reducing bacteria in human feces and their association with inflammatory bowel diseases. FEMS Microbiology Ecology. 2002;**40**(2):107-112

[57] Nishida A, Inoue R, Inatomi O, Bamba S, Naito Y, Andoh A. Gut

microbiota in the pathogenesis of inflammatory bowel disease. Clinical Journal of Gastroenterology [Internet]. 2018;**11**(1):1-10. DOI: 10.1007/s12328-017-0813-5

[58] Lloyd-Price J, Arze C, Ananthakrishnan AN, Schirmer M, Avila-Pacheco J, Poon TW, et al. Multi-omics of the gut microbial ecosystem in inflammatory bowel diseases. Nature. 2019;**569**(7758):655-662

[59] Rokkas T, Gisbert JP, Niv Y, O'Morain C. The association between helicobacter pylori infection and inflammatory bowel disease based on meta-analysis. United European Gastroenterology Journal. 2015;**3**(6):539-550

[60] Sokol H, Leducq V, Aschard H, Pham HP, Jegou S, Landman C, et al. Fungal microbiota dysbiosis in IBD. Gut. 2017;**66**(6):1039-1048

[61] Limon JJ, Tang J, Li D, Wolf AJ, Michelsen KS, Funari V, et al. Malassezia is associated with Crohn's disease and exacerbates colitis in mouse models. Cell Host & Microbe [Internet]. 2019;**25**(3):377-388.e6. DOI: 10.1016/j.chom.2019.01.007

[62] Zuo T, Ng SC. The gut microbiota in the pathogenesis and therapeutics of inflammatory bowel disease. Frontiers in Microbiology. 2018;**9**(Sep):1-13

[63] Norman JM, Handley SA, Baldridge MT, Droit L, Liu CY, Keller BC, et al. Disease-specific alterations in the enteric virome in inflammatory bowel disease. Cell [Internet]. 2015;**160**(3):447-460. DOI: 10.1016/j.cell.2015.01.002

[64] Pérez-Brocal V, García-López R, Vázquez-Castellanos JF, Nos P, Beltrán B, Latorre A, et al. Study of the viral and microbial communities associated with Crohn's disease: A metagenomic approach. Clinical and Translational Gastroenterology. 2013;**4**(6):e36. Published 13 Jun 2013. DOI:10.1038/ctg.2013.9

[65] Morgan XC, Tickle TL, Sokol H, Gevers D, Devaney KL, Ward DV, et al. Dysfunction of the intestinal microbiome in inflammatory bowel disease and treatment. Genome Biology. 2012;**13**(9):R79. Published 16 Apr 2012. DOI: 10.1186/gb-2012-13-9-r79

[66] Zhuang X, Tian Z, Li N, Mao R, Li X, Zhao M, et al. Gut microbiota profiles and microbial-based therapies in post-operative Crohn's disease: A systematic review. Frontiers in Medicine. Lausanne. 2021;**7**:615858. Published 28 Jan 2021. DOI: 10.3389/fmed.2020.615858

[67] Imhann F, Vich Vila A, Bonder MJ, Fu J, Di G, Visschedijk MC, et al. Interplay of host genetics and gut microbiota underlying the onset and clinical presentation of inflammatory bowel disease. Gut. 2018;**67**(1):108-119

[68] Hall AB, Yassour M, Sauk J, Garner A, Jiang X, Arthur T, et al. A novel Ruminococcus gnavus clade enriched in inflammatory bowel disease patients. Genome Medicine. 2017;**9**(1):1-12

[69] Seregin SS, Golovchenko N, Schaf B, Chen J, Pudlo NA, Mitchell J, et al. Erratum: NLRP6 protects il10−/− mice from colitis by limiting colonization of (Cell Reports (2017) 19(4) (733-745) (S2211124717304576) (10.1016/j.celrep.2017.03.080)). Cell Reports [Internet]. 2017;**19**(10):2174. DOI: 10.1016/j.celrep.2017.05.074

[70] Jarmakiewicz-Czaja S, Zielińska M, Sokal A, Filip R. Genetic and epigenetic etiology of inflammatory bowel disease: An update. Genes (Basel).

2022;**13**(12):2388. Published 16 Dec 2022. DOI: 10.3390/genes13122388

[71] Liu TC, Stappenbeck TS. Genetics and pathogenesis of inflammatory bowel disease. Annual Review of Pathology: Mechanisms of Disease. 2016;**11**(7351):127-148

[72] Zhen Y, Zhang H. NLRP3 inflammasome and inflammatory bowel disease. Frontiers in Immunology. 2019;**10**(Feb):1-10

[73] Zakrzewski M, Simms LA, Brown A, Appleyard M, Irwin J, Waddell N, et al. IL23R-protective coding variant promotes beneficial bacteria and diversity in the ileal microbiome in healthy individuals without inflammatory bowel disease. Journal of Crohn's & Colitis. 2019;**13**(4):451-461

[74] Krawiec P, Pawłowska-Kamieniak A, Pac-Kożuchowska E. Interleukin 10 and interleukin 10 receptor in paediatric inflammatory bowel disease: From bench to bedside lesson. Journal of Inflammation (United Kingdom). 2021;**18**(1):1-5

[75] Shouval D, Ouahed J, Biswas A, Al E. Interleukin 10 receptor signaling: Master regulator of intestinal mucosal homeostasis in mice and humans. Advances in Immunology. 2014;**122**(3):177-210

[76] Yilmaz B, Spalinger MR, Biedermann L, Franc Y, Fournier N, Rossel JB, et al. The presence of genetic risk variants within ptpn2 and ptpn22 is associated with intestinal microbiota alterations in Swiss IBD cohort patients. PLoS One. 2018;**13**(7):1-19

[77] Herbst S, Gutierrez MG. LRRK2 in infection: Friend or foe? ACS Infectious Diseases. 2019;**5**(6):809-815

[78] Caio G, Lungaro L, Caputo F, Zoli E, Giancola F, Chiarioni G, et al. Nutritional treatment in Crohn' s disease. Nutrients. 2021;**13**(5):1628

[79] Núñez-Sánchez MA, Melgar S, O'Donoghue K, Martínez-Sánchez MA, Fernández-Ruiz VE, Ferrer-Gómez M, et al. Crohn's disease, host–microbiota interactions, and immunonutrition: Dietary strategies targeting gut microbiome as novel therapeutic approaches. International Journal of Molecular Sciences. 2022;**23**(15)

[80] Guo X, Huang C, Xu J, Xu H, Liu L, Zhao H, et al. Gut microbiota is a potential biomarker in inflammatory bowel disease. Frontiers in Nutrition. 2022;**8**(January):1-11

[81] Ananthakrishnan AN. Microbiome-based biomarkers for ibd. Inflammatory Bowel Diseases. 2020;**26**(10):1463-1469

[82] Wills ES, Jonkers DMAE, Savelkoul PH, Masclee AA, Pierik MJ, Penders J. Fecal microbial composition of ulcerative colitis and Crohn's disease patients in remission and subsequent exacerbation. PLoS One. 2014;**9**(3):1-10

[83] Rehman A, Rausch P, Wang J, Skieceviciene J, Kiudelis G, Bhagalia K, et al. Geographical patterns of the standing and active human gut microbiome in health and IBD. Gut. 2016;**65**(2):238-248

[84] Lopez-Siles M, Martinez-Medina M, Busquets D, Sabat-Mir M, Duncan SH, Flint HJ, et al. Mucosa-associated Faecalibacterium prausnitzii and Escherichia coli co-abundance can distinguish irritable bowel syndrome and inflammatory bowel disease phenotypes. International Journal of Medical Microbiology [Internet]. 2014;**304**(3-4):464-475. DOI: 10.1016/j.ijmm.2014.02.009

[85] Ad B, Ag T, Ak A, Butterworth AD, Thomas AG, Akobeng AK. Probiotics for induction of remission in Crohn ' s disease (review) probiotics for induction of remission in Crohn' s disease. Library (London). 2008;**3**:3-5

[86] Abraham BP, Quigley EMM. Probiotics in inflammatory bowel disease. Gastroenterology Clinics of North America [Internet]. 2017;**46**(4):769-782. DOI: 10.1016/j.gtc.2017.08.003

[87] Fedorak RN, Feagan BG, Hotte N, Leddin D, Dieleman LA, Petrunia DM, et al. The probiotic vsl#3 has anti-inflammatory effects and could reduce endoscopic recurrence after surgery for Crohn's disease. Clinical Gastroenterology and Hepatology [Internet]. 2015;**13**(5):928-935.e2. DOI: 10.1016/j.cgh.2014.10.031

[88] Sornplang P, Piyadeatsoontorn S. Probiotic isolates from unconventional sources: A review. Journal of Animal Science and Technology [Internet]. 2016;**58**:1-11. DOI: 10.1186/s40781-016-0108-2

[89] Bazireh H, Shariati P, Azimzadeh Jamalkandi S, Ahmadi A, Boroumand MA. Isolation of novel probiotic lactobacillus and enterococcus strains from human salivary and fecal sources. Frontiers in Microbiology. 2020;**11**(December):1-12

[90] Schrezenmeir J, de Vrese M. Probiotics, prebiotics, and synbiotics—Approaching a definition. The American Journal of Clinical Nutrition. 2001; **73**(2 Suppl):361S-364S. DOI: 10.1093/ajcn/73.2.361s

[91] Oka A, Sartor B. Terapias basadas en microbios y dirigidas a microbios para enfermedades inflamatorias del intestino. Physiology & Behavior. 2020;**176**:139-148

[92] Belizário JE, Faintuch J. Microbiome and gut dysbiosis. Experientia. Supplementum. 2018;**109**:459-476

[93] van der Lelie D, Oka A, Taghavi S, Umeno J, Fan TJ, Merrell KE, et al. Rationally designed bacterial consortia to treat chronic immune-mediated colitis and restore intestinal homeostasis. Nature Communications. 2021;**12**(1):1-17

[94] Bernstein CN. Treatment of IBD: Where we are and where we are going. The American Journal of Gastroenterology [Internet]. 2015;**110**(1):114-126. DOI: 10.1038/ajg.2014.357

[95] Wu XW, Ji HZ, Wang FY. Meta-analysis of ciprofloxacin in treatment of Crohn's disease. Biomedical Reports. 2015;**3**(1):70-74

[96] Wang SL, Wang ZR, Yang CQ. Meta-analysis of broad-spectrum antibiotic therapy in patients with active inflammatory bowel disease. Experimental and Therapeutic Medicine. 2012;**4**(6):1051-1056

[97] Qv L, Mao S, Li Y, Zhang J, Li L. Roles of gut bacteriophages in the pathogenesis and treatment of inflammatory bowel disease. Frontiers in Cellular and Infection Microbiology. 2021;**11**(November):1-11

[98] Zhilu X, Xiangqian D, Keli Y, Caroline C, Jingwan Z, Yu L, et al. Association of adherent-invasive Escherichia coli with severe gut mucosal dysbiosis in Hong Kong Chinese population with Crohn's disease. Gut Microbes [Internet]. 2021;**13**(1):1-13. DOI: 10.1080/19490976.2021.1994833

[99] Galtier M, De Sordi L, Sivignon A, de Vallée A, Maura D, Neut C, et al. Bacteriophages targeting adherent

invasive Escherichia coli strains as a promising new treatment for Crohn's disease. Journal of Crohn's & Colitis. 2017;**11**(7):840-847

[100] Federici S, Kredo-Russo S, Valdés-Mas R, et al. Targeted suppression of human IBD-associated gut microbiota commensals by phage consortia for treatment of intestinal inflammation. Cell. 2022;**185**(16):2879-2898.e24. DOI: 10.1016/j.cell.2022.07.003

[101] Martín R, Chain F, Miquel S, Natividad JM, Sokol H, Verdu EF, et al. Effects in the use of a genetically engineered strain of Lactococcus lactis delivering in situ IL-10 as a therapy to treat low-grade colon inflammation. Human Vaccines & Immunotherapeutics. 2014;**10**(6):1611-1621

[102] Chiabai MJ, Almeida JF, De Azevedo MGD, Fernandes SS, Pereira VB, De Castro RJA, et al. Mucosal delivery of Lactococcus lactis carrying an anti-TNF scFv expression vector ameliorates experimental colitis in mice. BMC Biotechnology. 2019;**19**(1):1-12

[103] Namai F, Shigemori S, Ogita T, Sato T, Shimosato T. Microbial therapeutics for acute colitis based on genetically modified Lactococcus lactis hypersecreting IL-1Ra in mice. Experimental & Molecular Medicine [Internet]. 2020;**52**(9):1627-1636. DOI: 10.1038/s12276-020-00507-5

[104] Gevers D, Kugathasan S, Denson LA, Vázquez-Baeza Y, Van Treuren W, Ren B, et al. The treatment-naive microbiome in new-onset Crohn's disease. Cell Host & Microbe. 2014;**15**(3):382-392

[105] Saha S, Mara K, Pardi DS, Khanna S. Long-term safety of fecal microbiota transplantation for recurrent *Clostridioides difficile* infection. Gastroenterology [Internet]. 2021;**160**(6):1961-1969.e3. DOI: 10.1053/j.gastro.2021.01.010

[106] Du C, Luo Y, Walsh S, Grinspan A. Oral Fecal microbiota transplant capsules are safe and effective for recurrent *Clostridioides difficil*e infection: A systematic review and meta-analysis. Journal of Clinical Gastroenterology. 2021;**55**(4):300-308. DOI: 10.1097/MCG.0000000000001495

Chapter 3

Difficulties in the Differential Diagnosis of Crohn's Disease

Gulustan H. Babayeva, Gunay V. Asadova, Jamal S. Musayev, Umud R. Mahmudov, Farid V. Quliyev and Aychin I. Hasanova

Abstract

Currently, the main difficulty in the accurate diagnosis of inflammatory bowel disease (IBD) is associated with the high prevalence of infectious, allergic and autoimmune diseases leading to intestinal lesions mimicking IBD. In geographical regions where there is endemicity for certain infections, in particular tuberculosis, timely verification of the diagnoses of ulcerative colitis (UC) and Crohn's disease (CD) is a serious problem. Some infectious, allergic and autoimmune pathologies can not only imitate the clinical and endoscopic picture of IBD, but also complicate the course of an existing IBD, as a result of which there is resistance to the prescribed basic therapy in patients with UC and CD. Unfortunately, the complexity and limited possibilities of diagnostic methods can often be the reason for the belated establishment of an accurate diagnosis. Thus, in all these diseases, the main fecal markers for verifying the diagnosis of IBD, fecal calprotectin and lactoferrin, often have elevated values.

Keywords: inflammatory bowel disease, infectious colitis, tuberculosis, Behçet's disease, autoimmune diseases, vasculitis

1. Introduction

At the turn of the twenty-first century, due to a local increase in the incidence of inflammatory bowel diseases, they have become a global medical and social problem. If by the end of 2017 the highest prevalence rates were in Europe (ulcerative colitis 505 per 100,000 in Norway; Crohn's disease 322 per 100,000 in Germany) and North America (ulcerative colitis 286 per 100,000 in the USA; Crohn's disease 319 per 100,000 in Canada), by the end of 2019, the prevalence of inflammatory bowel disease exceeded 0.3% of the total population in many other regions of the Earth. As of April 2020, over 2 million people in North America, 3.2 million in Europe, and over 10 million worldwide have IBD. Despite the fact that the incidence in developed Western countries is stabilizing, the burden of costs associated with solving emerging problems remains high [1, 2].

Inflammatory bowel diseases are immune-mediated diseases, due to which "cross-overs" with various autoimmune, infectious, proliferative diseases are quite common.

Considering the growing incidence of IBD, the high prevalence of opportunistic (including intestinal) infections and "overlap syndromes" with autoimmune, and currently with allergic pathologies, as well as the lack of a single diagnostic "gold" standard, clinicians are faced with a large number of problems.

For the diagnosis of IBD, several world ducts have been adopted today, and in all endoscopy with pathomorphological examination, it is accepted as a mandatory criterion in diagnostic algorithms for verifying the diagnoses of ulcerative colitis, Crohn's disease, microscopic and undifferentiated colitis.

2. Pathologies, mimicking IBD

2.1 IBD mimics

Infectious		**Non-infectious**
Small intestine/terminal ileum	*Colon*	*Granulomas present* • Sarcoidosis, small vessel vasculitides • Hermansky-Pudlak syndrome • CVID (common variable immunodeficiency) *Ulcer in mouth and small/large intestine* • Behcet's disease *Colon inflammation* • Diverticulitis • SCAD (segmental colitis associated with diverticulosis) • Drug induced colitis (NSAIDs, immunotherapy) • Ischemic colitis • SRUS (solitary rectal ulcer syndrome) *Non-specific mucosal changes without chronic inflammation* • IBS (irritable bowel syndrome) • Cancer (adenocarcinomas, GL lymphomas, others)
Bacterial • Tuberculosis • Yersinia • Salmonella *Fungal* • Histoplazma • Coccidioides	*Bacterial* • *C. difficile* • *Salmonella* • *Shigella* • *E. coli* • *Campylobacter* • Aeromonas *Parasitic* • Amebiasis (*E. histolytica*) *Viral* • CMV	

3. Intestinal tuberculosis (ITB)

Diagnosis of IBD in regions where tuberculosis (TB) is common is a major diagnostic challenge. This is especially true for Crohn's disease, since CD and ITB are chronic granulomatous diseases, quite often with overlapping endoscopic, pathomorphological, radiological, and clinical findings. The similarity in clinical manifestations of these two diseases, as well as the absence of specific laboratory markers of intestinal tuberculosis, may possibly explain the high misdiagnosis rates, which range from 50 to 70% [3]. Misdiagnosis and subsequent treatment can lead to undesirable consequences. For this reason, many clinical studies have examined the role of endoscopy (colonoscopy), pathology, clinical manifestations, quantiferon test (IGRA), polymerase chain reaction (PCR) detection of *Mycobacterium tuberculosis*, and comprehensive scoring systems in differentiating between ITB and CD.

The symptoms and signs of abdominal tuberculosis are nonspecific and may closely resemble CD and other gastrointestinal pathologies. TB can be confused with cancer of the respective areas. Intestinal TB may be detected in asymptomatic patients who have had a colonoscopy for other reasons. Pain is the most common presentation, in approximately 85% of patients, weight loss in 66%, fever in 35–50%, and diarrhea in 20% of patients. Systemic manifestations (subfebrile temperature, fever in the evening, lethargy, malaise, night sweats and weight loss) can be detected in 30% of patients. This is more often observed with tuberculous ascitic-type peritonitis and ulcerative lesions of the intestine. Abdominal tenderness occurs in most patients, and a mass in the abdomen, usually in the right lower quadrant, in 25 to 50% of patients. Malabsorption is observed in 21–75% of cases [4–6]. Acute abdomen: In developing countries, extrapulmonary (abdominal) TB can often present as an acute abdominal process during emergency surgery such as perforation and intestinal obstruction [4–6]. Ascites can be caused by peritoneal tuberculosis or result from hepatic, malignant, cardiac, renal or other infectious diseases [22]. Peritoneal tuberculosis with ascites may occur with less pain and complication than purulent peritonitis with perforation. "Cocoon" of the abdominal cavity–an unusual form of tuberculosis of the abdominal cavity–is characterized by the formation of a fibrous membrane sac around the loops of the small intestine. While conservative treatment with antituberculous therapy (ATT) may suffice for some patients, while other patients who do not respond to treatment require surgical intervention [5, 6]. Anorectal TB may present as a stricture, anal fistula, or anal fissure.

Colonoscopy can be useful for differential diagnosis if it is performed by a doctor who knows the features of these pathologies. A study in Korea in 2006 found that the diagnosis of ITB or CD by colonoscopy was correct in 87.5% of patients (77/88), incorrect in 8.0% of patients (7/88), and was considered indeterminate in 4.5% of patients (4/88) [4]. In another study, including 122 cases of ITB and 130 cases of CD, a mathematical regression equation was developed according to endoscopic parameters: rectal involvement, longitudinal ulcers, transverse ulcers, cobblestone syndrome, fixed open ileocecal valve (**Figure 1a** and **b**) [2, 5].

The presence of macroscopic lesions along with microscopic detection of inflammatory infiltration in the terminal ileum often leads the gastroenterologist to the diagnosis of Crohn's disease (CD).

In CD, pathomorphological diagnosis is problematic due to the lack of specific microscopic features and discrete lesions. The Singapore study assessed the baseline features of mucosal biopsy in 25 CD patients, 3 patients with ITB, and 2 cases of colitis associated with diverticular disease. Granulomas were observed in 10 of 41 CD biopsies and in all 5 other biopsies. Small, firm, well-circumscribed granulomas are characteristic of CD compared with large coalesced granulomas in tuberculosis. Cellular,

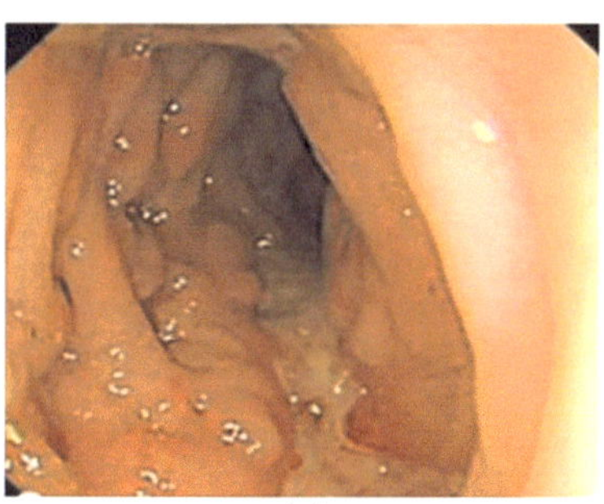

(a)

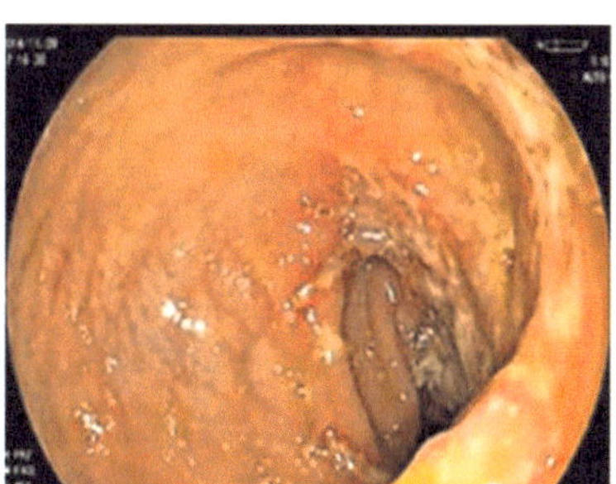

(b)

Figure 1.
Endoscopic picture of intestinal lesions in CD and ITB [5]. (a) typical longitudinal ulcers in a patient with CD. (b) typical transverse ulcers in a patient with ITB.

pseudopyloric and Paneth's metaplasia was observed only in CD (2/25) [7]. Due to the low sensitivity of standard biopsy sampling, which is limited to the mucosa only and involves the submucosal layer, it is difficult to make an accurate diagnosis based on the histology of the biopsy. To date, the role of the quantiferon test (IGRA) in differentiating ITB from CD has been sufficiently studied. A systematic review with a meta-analysis of IGRA accuracy was published in 2014 [3]. The sensitivity, specificity, positive predictive value, and negative predictive value of the tests in the 8 studies averaged 81, 85, 78, and 87%, respectively. In conditions of high incidence of tuberculosis, when latent infection is widespread, a positive result of the quantiferon test does not make it possible to distinguish between active and latent tuberculosis [8]. However, in TB endemic regions, this test is necessary to rule out TB in IBD, as evidenced by a high negative predictive value (94.2%) [9]. PCR analysis also helps differentiate TB from CD by detecting M. tuberculosis DNA in biopsy or stool specimens. The reported sensitivity and specificity of TB-PCR mucosal biopsy were 64.1% and 100%, respectively [10]. However, one must be aware of the possibility of false positive or negative results (primer not specific enough or limited amount of tissue available in mucosal biopsy specimens). M. tuberculosis DNA has also been reported to be found in mucus and fecal samples of some CD patients due to the presence of latent tuberculosis [10–12].

Computed tomography (CT) enterography also plays a role in disease differentiation. Segmental involvement, comb sign, changes in fibro-adipose tissue, moderate wall thickening, and asymmetric distribution are significantly more common in CD patients than in patients with ITB [13]. The combination of CT enterography with endoscopy data increases the accuracy of diagnosing CD and/or ITB from 66.7 to 95.2% [14]. In addition, concurrent active pulmonary tuberculosis detected by computed tomography may add value to the diagnosis of ITB.

Differentiation between CD and ITB is the most difficult, as there are cases of crossover options. In this case, the practitioner needs to remember the differential features of CD and ITB (see **Table 1**).

Peculiarities	**CD**	**ITB**
Clinical:	Specific (disease of the perianal region)	
Perianal lesion		Rarely Peritoneal involvement with ascites (but this is often absent and not very discriminatory)
Blood in stool	Present	Rarely
Endoscopy:	$\geq$ 4 segments	< 4 segments
Lesions		
Ulcer shape	Longitudinal ulcers Aphthoid ulceration Cobblestones	Transverse ulcers, nodules, scars, strictures of short segments
Ileocecal valve disease	Rarely Long segment of the ileum with preservation of the ileocecal valve	Specific The ileocecal valve is almost always affected - a fixed, patulous ileocecal valve is a very typical finding in ITB
Quantiferon test	Negative PCR and tissue culture for TB	Positive tissue TB PCR and culture

Peculiarities	CD	ITB
		Positive IGRA and/or PPD test result
Active pulmonary TIB (Chest X-ray/CT)	Negative	Specific
CT enterography:	Specific	Less specific
Multisegmental lesion		
Sigmoid/rectal lesion	Specific	Less specific
Asymmetric lesions	Specific	Less specific
"Comb" symptom	Specific	Less specific
Fibro-fatty changes	Specific	Less specific
Radiographic features and radiological signs:	long segment strictures, multi-site involvement, ridge sign, perianal disease.	short strictures, deformed ileocecal valve, lymphadenopathy with hypodense centers, thickened peritoneum
Histology of the biopsy	Granulomas (noncaseating, small, losses and infrequent); focally enhanced colitis; loss of mucosal architecture is present even at a distance from granulomas	Granulomas (caseous, large, confluent and many others); architectural mucosal loss only close to granuloma; protruding submucosal inflammation
Focal chronic inflammation	Specific	Less specific
Granuloma	Solitary, <400 μm, noncaseating	Sticky, ≥400 μm, caseous
Features of the course of the disease	Younger age Relapses and remissions Shorter duration of symptoms Intestinal fistulas Extraintestinal manifestations of CD (although TB involvement of the joints of the lower extremities, skin, eyes, and liver may mimic extraintestinal CD)	Chronic, continuous course of the disease High temperature (>38.5 °C) without intra-abdominal abscess (although fever is seen in both CD and ITB)

Table 1.
Clinical, endoscopic, laboratory, radiological, histological features and features of the course of the disease of CD and 1 TB [14–18].

4. Yersiniosis, histioplasmosis, granulomatous enterocolitis

The presence of macroscopic lesions along with microscopic detection of inflammatory infiltration in the terminal ileum often leads the clinician to the diagnosis of Crohn's disease. However, some of these cases may actually be Yersinia spp. infection, with or without CD, which can be easily diagnosed. John K. Triantafillidis et al. recommended testing serum antibodies against YOP antigens in all patients with endoscopic and histological evidence of terminal ileitis to identify yersiniosis with or without terminal ileal CD [19, 20].

In recent years, inflammatory lesions of the terminal ileum mucosa have been increasingly recognized due to easy endoscopic access. Moreover, the histological finding of inflammation in symptomatic individuals prompted endoscopists to hastily diagnose Crohn's disease in the absence of a recent history of drug use or viral infection. However, a number of these cases may actually correspond to Yersinia infection, as tests for serum antibodies against Yersinia outer protein (YOP) antigens are not usually performed. Thus, it is reasonable to assume that some cases characterized as CD, especially those of mild severity, are in fact cases of yersiniosis that resolve spontaneously or are followed by treatment with ciprofloxacin, the antibiotic commonly used by most gastroenterologists worldwide in patients with CD. It is not known whether the coexistence of Yersinia infection and CD in the same patient increases the severity of the underlying enteropathy. In addition, the ability of Yersinia to survive in natural specimens and thrive at low temperatures means that the true contribution of this pathogen to disease may be underestimated.

YE has been isolated from patients in many parts of the world, but appears to be predominantly found in cooler climates, including northern Europe, Scandinavia, and Japan. The prevalence of infection is higher from November to January. In the US, YE infection accounts for 5% of intestinal infections among children under 5 years of age. Isolation of YE in developing countries is rare [21]. YE is transmitted to humans through water, food, soil and animals. YE has also been isolated from flies found in piggeries and farm kitchens, suggesting that arthropod/insect vectors may contribute to animal-to-human transmission of Yersinia [22]. The infection is transmitted mainly by the fecal-oral route. Consumption of pork (especially undercooked) or raw pork products is a cause of yersiniosis. Outbreaks from drinking water contaminated with this pathogen have also been reported. There are reports of cases of transmission from an infected pet and through transfused blood products. It is important to emphasize that infected people can pass YE in their stool for at least 90 days after the symptoms have disappeared.

Zadernowskaya et al. have shown that blue cheese may be a suitable growth medium for YE. Given the fact that YE can grow under cold conditions, they can pose a real threat to human health [23]. In patients diagnosed with TI, an infectious cause can be found in a third of cases; including Yersinia spp., CD can also be demonstrated in 12.1% of patients [24]. Taking into account these two critical conditions, namely Yersinia infection and CD, it can be concluded that TI can occur under three conditions: TI due to Yersinia infection, TI due to CD, and TI due to the coexistence of Yersinia infection with CD. Yersinia species are often found in small amounts in the terminal ileum in both healthy individuals and patients with TI. According to the latest data, Y. infection was detected in CD tissues no more often than in tissues of inflammatory and non-inflammatory control [25]. However, in a study to determine the seroprevalence of anti-Yersinia antibodies in 750 healthy Austrians using the recomBlot Yersinia Western blot kit, an overall seroprevalence of 29.7% was found. Seroprevalence increased significantly with age: from 24.7% in the group of people aged 19 to 24 years to 38.5% in the group of people over 44 years of age. This high seroprevalence contrasts with the small number of reported cases suggesting a subclinical or mild infection [26]. Knösel et al. showed that although several potential pathogens can be detected in tissue samples from CD patients, these pathogens can also be detected in controls, suggesting that many infectious pathogens may be associated with CD, but they are not necessarily cause [27]. In a subsequent study of 44 Crohn's disease patients tested for Yersinia infection, a significant proportion of patients (39%) were positive [28]. Finally, a German study found an average annual incidence of yersiniosis of 7.2/100,000 population, with a higher incidence found in children under 5 years of age. About 90% of infections occurred within the country. The predominant serotype was O:3 [29]. Intestinal yersiniosis can present with TI, enteritis, mesenteric lymphadenitis, pseudoappendicitis, and septicemia. The incubation period is usually 4 to 6 days (1 to 14 days). Acute infection may result in mucosal ulceration (usually in the terminal ileum and rarely in the ascending colon), necrotic Peyer's patches, and mesenteric lymph node enlargement. Symptoms include diarrhea or bloody stools, abdominal pain, and fever. The duration of diarrhea in acute yersiniosis can be from 12 to 22 days. The infection usually resolves within a few weeks with or without antibiotics. However, complications such as reactive arthritis can appear 1–4 weeks after infection, with an increased risk if a person tests positive for the MHC HLA-B27 allele [30].

Yersiniosis is difficult to distinguish from other causes of acute diarrhea. Localization of pain in the right hypochondrium can be a diagnostic sign of yersiniosis. Sepsis has been described in patients who are immunocompromised or in a state of iron overload. Acute yersiniosis can also mimic appendicitis (pseudo-appendicitis), which presents with right lower quadrant pain, fever, vomiting, elevated white blood cells, and diarrhea. Emergency surgery demonstrates inflammation of the terminal ileum and mesenteric lymph nodes with a normal appendix [31]. In a study aimed at elucidating the long-term prognosis in patients with TI, it was found that isolated acute TI detected during diagnostic ileocolonoscopy rarely leads to a definitive diagnosis of CD (4.6%) and that only the presence of strictures on a transverse section can predict the development of celiac disease [32]. In patients with Yersinia infection and symptoms suggestive of acute appendicitis, abdominal MRI may show evidence of TI with a normal appendix. Further examination in these cases may reveal Yersinia infection [33]. Yersinia infection can also present with liver or spleen abscesses [34], bacteremia, septic arthritis [35] or aseptic skin abscesses [36].

Yersinia infection may precede the diagnosis of CD. Zippi et al. described a patient with mesenteric adenitis due to yersiniosis who was subsequently diagnosed with CD [37]. Whether the presence of microorganisms is an epiphenomenon or actually a contributing factor to the pathogenesis of CD is currently unknown. Homewood et al. [38] described another case of terminal ileitis caused by YP infection. The patient was subsequently diagnosed with CD [39–41]. In addition, YE DNA was found in the histology of colonic and mesenteric lymph node resections in a number of CD cases. In a related study, the incidence of inflammatory bowel disease was found to be higher in anti-YE serum antibody-positive patients than in antibody-negative group [42]. The incidence of reactive arthritis following YE infection varies across countries. The knee and ankle joints are most commonly affected. In most cases, two to four joints are involved sequentially and asymmetrically over a period of several days to 2 weeks. In two-thirds of cases, acute arthritis persists for 1 to 4 months. Chronic joint disease or ankylosing spondylitis is rare. Gastrointestinal complications include intestinal perforation, peritonitis, ulcerative ileitis and colitis, intussusception, paralytic ileus, cholangitis, mesenteric vein thrombosis, toxic megacolon, liver and spleen abscesses, liver failure, and small bowel necrosis, and extraintestinal complications include septicemia, renal failure, abscess, osteomyelitis, lung abscess, endocarditis, purulent lymphadenitis, skin infection, fungal aneurysm, myocarditis and glomerulonephritis.

Diagnosis depends on a detailed history, physical examination, laboratory findings, and imaging. The diagnosis can also be confirmed by positive cultures obtained from mesenteric lymph nodes, pharyngeal exudate, peritoneal fluid, or blood. Polymerase chain reaction and immunofluorescent analysis have been developed. Endoscopy and imaging studies (ultrasound or CT) are often required to determine whether a patient has appendicitis or pseudo-appendicitis. Serological tests, including ELISA assays and immunoblotting for the detection of IgG, IgA, and IgM, are used in many countries.

The detection of antibodies against YOP has made a significant contribution to the diagnostic arsenal. Antibodies against the microorganism are produced shortly after infection and persist for a long period of time. Antibody levels begin to rise during the first week of illness, peak in the second week, and then return to normal within 3 to 6 months. However, antibodies can remain detectable for several years. Polymerase chain reaction is now suspected in patients with suspected terminal ileitis as culture-based diagnostics of Y. infection are gradually being replaced by molecular tests. DNA microarray for pathogenic organisms, a relatively new technique that is used to identify several genes of various types of pathogens, has been used to diagnose Y. infection. Endoscopy is very useful in identifying mucosal lesions in the terminal ileum and obtaining a biopsy to assess the extent and type of inflammation. Results can vary and in most cases are relatively non-specific. Typically, in patients with YE infection, aphthoid ulcers may be found in the caecum, and small rounded elevations and ulcers may be demonstrated in the terminal ileum, and exudates may be present; the left side of the colon is usually not affected. In one study of eight patients, with fecal isolation of Yersinia and serum anti-Yersinia antibodies, all had terminal ileum involvement followed by involvement of the ileocecal valve and caecum and, to a lesser extent, the ascending colon [43]. The main endoscopic findings were round or oval elevations with or without ulcers in the terminal ileum. However, small ulcers have also been found in the ileocecal valve as well as in the caecum [43]. Interestingly, these endoscopic findings were visible 5 weeks after symptom onset.

Histologic evidence of Yersinia infection is not pathognomonic and usually indicates only acute and/or chronic inflammation. Focal villous atrophy and crypt hyperplasia with mixed acute and chronic inflammation and focal neutrophilic cryptitis, as well as epithelial cell granulomas consisting of histiocytes and small T-lymphocytes and plasma monocytes with suppurative centers have been reported [41, 44]. Whereas small bowel infection caused by yersiniosis results in the formation of necrotizing granulomas, small bowel adenoviral lesions cause marked lymphoid hyperplasia, which in turn can lead to obstructive or intussusception ileus [45]. In biopsy material, because necrotizing granulomas are usually located deep. Adenovirus affects more epithelial cells.

In immunosuppressed patients, a number of other pathogens can be detected, for example, cryptococcal enteritis, histoplasmosis.

Histoplasmosis is the most common endemic pathology [46]. Immunosuppressive status increases the risk of developing severe disease, but gastrointestinal histoplasmosis can occur in immunocompetent patients and mimic Crohn's disease. Lamps and all [46] studied 56 biopsies stained with silver and H&E from 52 patients. In 43% of patients, the disease manifested itself more with signs of gastrointestinal damage than with signs of lung damage. Grossly, changes in the gastrointestinal tract were represented by ulcers (49%), nodules (21%), bleeding (13%), obstructive growths (6%), and normal mucosa (23%). Microscopic changes included diffuse lymphohistiocytic infiltration (83%), ulceration (45%), lymphohistiocytic nodules (25%) or minimal inflammatory response (15%), and very rarely regular granulomas (8.5%). The most common finding in the liver was lymphohistiocytic infiltration in the region of the portal tracts. Focal granulomas in the liver were observed in less than 20% of cases. In these groups, about half of the patients were immunocompetent, which highlights the need to consider the possibility of developing this pathology before making a diagnosis of Crohn's disease. The differential diagnosis of granulomatous enterocolitis includes enterocolitis, which develops in a number of diseases accompanied by the formation of granulomas in other organs. Some infectious diseases are relatively specific for the gastrointestinal tract, for example, the above-mentioned yersiniosis, some variants of salmonellosis. The granulomatous process in yersiniosis is centered around Peyer's patches.

Some forms of immunodeficiency can also lead to the development of granulomatous colitis. Chronic granulomatous disease is a hereditary disorder manifested by immunodeficiency caused by a mutation in any of the genes encoding various subunits of the superoxide-forming phagocytic NADPH oxidase system, which is responsible for an oxidative burst that leads to the death of microorganisms. Chronic granulomatous disease can affect the gastrointestinal tract in about a third of patients and is manifested by a pronounced accumulation of macrophages and eosinophils. Granulomas, if present, are usually irregularly shaped and the macrophages are pigmented. Rare cases of common variable immunodeficiency are also characterized by the formation of granulomas, the hallmark of common variable immunodeficiency is the absence of plasma cells in its own plastic and apoptosis. If other granulomatous lesions are excluded, sarcoidosis, which is rare in the lower gastrointestinal tract, should be considered.

Cytomegalovirus infection in the small intestine has the same manifestations as in any other localization.

Escherichia coli is an exception among infectious colitis, as it leads to ischemic colitis. In such cases, neutrophils with crypt abscesses are detected, often localized in the upper half of the mucous membrane, and pronounced neutrophils in the lamina propria of the mucous membrane. Basal plasmacytosis, detected in inflammatory bowel diseases, is absent, the structure of the glands remains normal. Erosions and edema of the lamina propria are found. The disease stops on its own, its course correlates with what bacteria are found in the fecal masses. As the self-limiting colitis subsides (which often occurs by the time of biopsy), biopsy specimens show reactive epithelial changes, but the shape of the crypts remains unchanged. With regard to specific pathogens affecting the colon, bacterial colitis is often caused by *Campylobacter* spp. or Aeromonas spp., but bacteriological and cultural examination of feces is required to accurately determine the pathogen. In cases of immunodeficiency, cytomegalovirus and various parasites may be found in the colon. Colon biopsies show schistosome and Strongyloides eggs. In patients with HIV, biopsy specimens show characteristic giant cell colitis.

Colon spirochetosis is a characteristic condition in which the surface of the colon is lined with numerous organisms stained using the Warthin-Starry method. The disease is manifested by abdominal pain, appendicitis, chronic diarrhea, and in some cases rectal bleeding. In most cases, spirochetosis is an incidental finding that is not accompanied by overt clinical manifestations. On endoscopic examination, the mucosa may appear completely normal, or there may be areas of ulceration, erosion, edema, and/or hyperemia of the mucosa. In most cases, the causative agents of spirochetosis are the anaerobic intestinal spirochetes *Brachyspira aalborgi* and *Brachyspira pilosicoli*. *B. pilosicoli* colonizes the intestinal tract of many animals, especially pigs, and is found in the feces of 30% of people in developing countries.

5. Behçet's disease

Behçet's disease (BD) is a chronic multisystem inflammatory disease characterized by recurrent oral and/or genital aphthous ulcers and may be complicated by thrombotic and/or inflammatory lesions of the skin, eyes, joints, gastrointestinal tract, and/

or CNS. The disease is most common in East Asia and in the countries of the Mediterranean basin. The incidence of gastrointestinal involvement in Behcet's disease varies and is 2.8% in patients in Turkey, 32% in Taiwan, 37–43% in the United States, and 50–60% in Japan [47].

Intestinal BD and inflammatory bowel disease share a considerable number of genetic backgrounds, pathogenesis, and clinical features. Moreover, current therapeutic strategies for intestinal BD have many similarities to those of IBD. Some experts classify the two diseases as the same category of a single disease or as different spectrums of the same disease; others regard them as totally different diseases (see **Table 2**) [48].

In 1990, the International Study Group (ISG) for BD established a set of diagnostic criteria [48]. The ISG criteria for BD are not a perfect tool and cannot replace clinical judgment, but they are helpful for reminding clinicians of the most important diagnostic features of BD [48]. However, the ISG criteria for BD do not include intestinal symptoms.

	Similarities	Distinctions
Genetics	Interleukin (IL)-10 and the IL-23R-IL-12RB2 loci	Human leukocyte antigen-B51 allele MHC class I related gene A
Immunology	Activation of innate and adaptive immune system Increased Th1, Th17, CD4+ and CD8+ T cell, and γδ + T cell activities Increased Th1-type cytokines The rate of anti-Saccharomyces cerevisiae antibodies detection is remarkably higher Bacterial contribution to the disease development	Serum anti-Herpes simplex virus-1 antibodies in the patients with BD were significantly higher than controls Heat shock protein (HSP) stimulate γδ + T cells in BD patients because of homology between Streptococcus sanguis and human HSP Anti-endothelial cell antibody
Clinical findings	Wide variation of abdominal symptoms from mild discomfort to hematochezia Similar extra-intestinal manifestations	Rare anorectal involvement in intestinal BD Possible ischemic damage from vasculitis
Endoscopic findings	Segmental involvement Various type of ulcerations are able to seen Grossly normal looking intervening mucosa Mucosal healing is closely related with favorable clinical course	Fewer number of lesion Large size of ulceration Round or oval shaped ulceration Relatively more discrete and elevated border of ulceration
Histologic findings	Non-specific inflammation (lymphocytic or neutrophilic infiltrations)	Vasculitis can be seen Absence of non-caseating granuloma
Disease activity index	Concordance with clinical disease activity Discordance with endoscopic disease activity	Highly weighted general condition of patient and abdominal pain Less concern for laboratory test and diarrhea
Treatment	5-amino-salicylates/sulfasalazine, corticosteroids, thiopurines, thalidomide, and biologic agents are used for intestinal lesion	Concomitant use of medications for systemic BD is frequent
Prognosis	Similar admission, operation, and post-operative recurrence rate	Higher cumulative rate in use of corticosteroids and immunomodulators

Table 2.
Similarities and distinctions of intestinal Behçet's disease (BD) with Crohn's disease [48].

Based on the ISG criteria, the diagnosis is clinically verifiable and includes recurrent oral aphthae (≥3 recurrences per year) (see **Figure 2**) plus any 2 of the following: genital aphthae (see **Figure 3**), ocular lesions, skin lesions and/or a positive pattern test [49].

Although the ileocecal region is most commonly affected in intestinal BD, other regions of the GI system may also be involved, including the esophagus, stomach, duodenum, jejunum, and colon (see **Table 3**) [50].

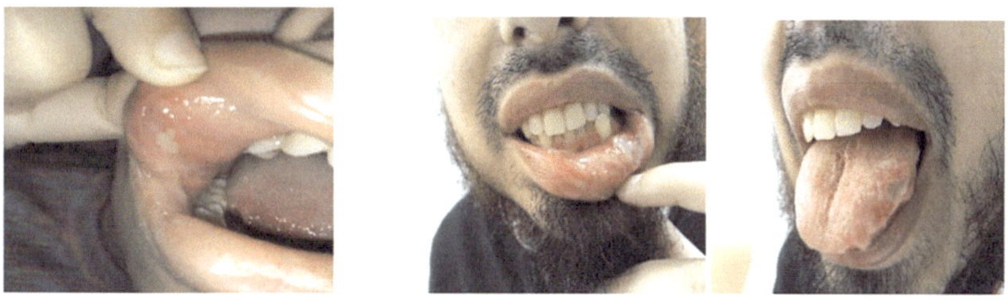

(a) (b)

Figure 2.
Oral lesions in Behçet's disease (unpublished materials from the authors' archives (Babayeva G.H.)). (a) the patient is 18 years old (b) the patient is 31 years old.

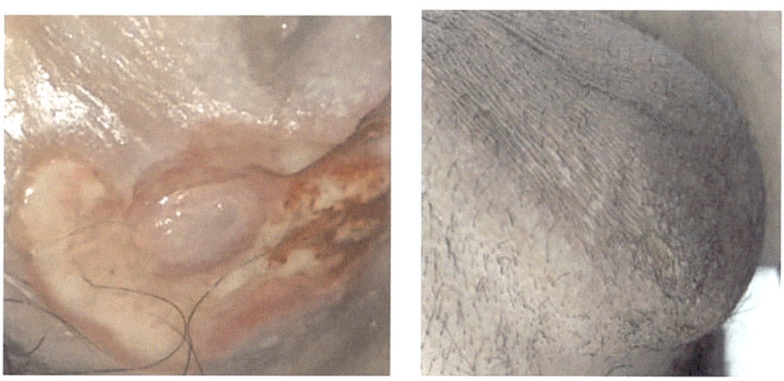

(a) (b)

Figure 3.
Genital lesions in Behcet's disease (unpublished materials from the authors' archives (Babayeva G.H.)). (a) 18-year-old patient (b) 31-year-old patient, signs of genital ulcers.

Anatomie site(s)	Gastrointestinal manifestation(s)
Esophagus	Ulcers,* esophagitis, fistulae, strictures, varices
Stomach, small intestine, colon	Ulcers*
Anal/rectal region	Ulcers,* fistulae, abscesses, proctitis, fissures
Liver	Budd-Chiari syndrome (acute, subacute, or chronic), fatty liver disease, hepatomegaly, congestion, cirrhosis
Spleen	Splenomegaly, congestion
Pancreas	Acute pancreatitis

**Ulcers are typically round, deep, and well demarcated, regardless of their location.*

Table 3.
Gastrointestinal manifestations of Behçet Disease (Adapted from Bayraktar Y, Ozaslan E, Van Thiel DH) [50].

In 2020, the Japanese Society of Gastroenterology published "Evidence-based diagnosis and clinical practice guidelines for intestinal Behcet's disease 2020 edited by Intractable Diseases, the Health and Labor Sciences Research Grants" [51].

Typically, volcano-shaped ulcers (see **Figure 4**) around the ileocecal region, right lower abdominal pain, and bloody stool are observed in intestinal BD (see **Figure 5**). Occasionally, patients experience severe abdominal symptoms as a result of ileus, perforation/penetration, and massive hemorrhage [52]. Intestinal BD is suspected when patients with BD (including suspected BD) present with these symptoms [53]. However, it is sometimes difficult to diagnose patients who have not been diagnosed with BD and do not present these symptoms. Differential diagnosis from other diseases, such as CD, is established while considering the presence/absence of local symptoms of BD, including recurring oral aphthae [52, 53].

The intestinal phenotype of BD is characterized by gastrointestinal manifestations that include, but are not limited to, chronic abdominal pain, diarrhea, gastrointestinal bleeding, mucosal ulceration, and intestinal perforation. Two forms of intestinal manifestations of Behcet's disease can be distinguished: mucosal ulcers resulting from neutrophilic infiltrates, which can mimic IBD, and intestinal ischemia and infarcts due to large vessel vasculitis, especially mesenteric [54]. To date, there is no consensus in the world regarding the diagnosis of this phenotype of BD.

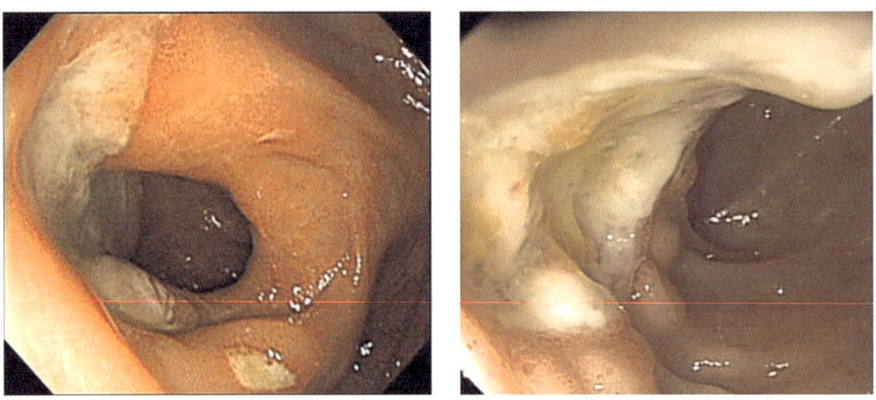

Figure 4.
Typical ileocecal ulcer in a patient with Behcet's disease.

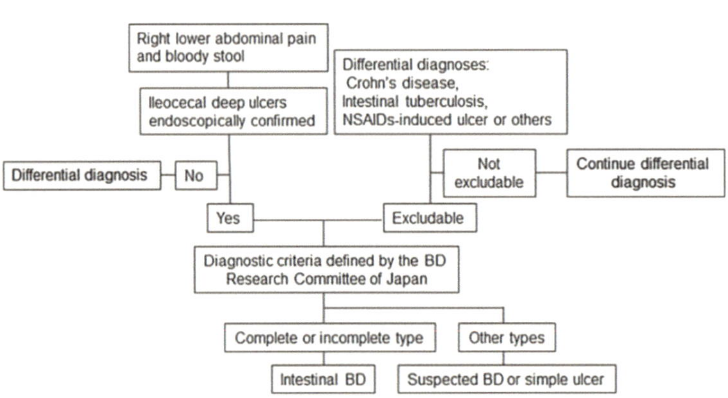

Figure 5.
Algorithm for a definite diagnosis of intestinal BD.

In one study, up to 50% of BD patients with intestinal lesions required surgical interventions associated with intestinal perforation, gastrointestinal bleeding, and fistula formation [55]. Any part of the gastrointestinal tract can be involved in the pathological process, most often the terminal ileum and the ileocecal intestine. Three types of ulcers have been described in the colon: volcanic, geographic, and aphthous. Volcanic ulcers have the highest risk of perforation, especially in patients younger than 25 years of age. Rectal and/or anal involvement is rare.

When examining biopsies of the superficial layers of the mucosa, only nonspecific changes are found: signs of chronic active inflammation of the mucosa, changes in architectonics with possible ulceration, resembling inflammatory bowel diseases. The most important diagnostic feature is characteristic vasculitis, which is often only possible to detect when studying the surgical material of the resected intestine.

The intestinal phenotype of BD and IBD has a sufficient number of similarities, in particular: the onset of the disease occurs at a young age, nonspecific gastrointestinal symptoms and similar extraintestinal manifestations, as well as a chronically relapsing course of the disease are noted. The similarity of the two diseases and the lack of reliable diagnostic criteria make differentiation difficult.

One retrospective study showed that extraintestinal systemic manifestations and characteristic endoscopic features such as distribution, size, and type of ulcer may contribute to the differential diagnosis of the intestinal phenotype of BD from CD [56]. Focal lesions, deformity of the ileocecal valve, solitary and large ulcers (ulcer size >2 sm), ulcer tendency to merge around the circumference were more frequent in patients with the intestinal form of BD (**Figure 6**) [2, 5, 8]. A Korean study proposed a new and simple diagnostic criterion based on two aspects: colonoscopy findings and extraintestinal manifestations [57]. This added additional features, especially in patients with ileocolonic ulcers, who do not fully meet the diagnostic criteria for systemic BD [58]. The clinical and endoscopic features of CD and BD are listed in **Table 4**, **Table 5** and **Figure 7**.

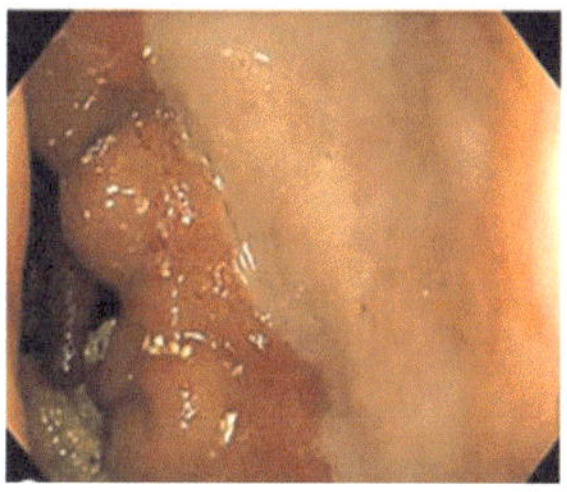

Figure 6.
Endoscopic image of the lesion of the ileocecal region in Behcet's disease (single, rounded, large ulcers) [5].

Peculiarities	CD	BD
Clinical:		
Abdominal pain	Usually associated with intestinal obstruction	Severe pain without signs of intestinal obstruction
Ulcers in the oral cavity (see **Figure 2**)	Specific	≥3/year, painful
Ulcers in the genital area (see **Figure 3**)	Not specific	Present

Peculiarities	**CD**	**BD**
Endoscopic: (See **Figures 4** and **6**)	Longitudinal	Round
Ulcer shape		
Spreading	Segmental	Focal, solitary
Areas involved	Ileocecal	Ileocecal

Table 4.
Clinical and endoscopic features of Crohn's disease and Behçet's disease.

	Behçet's Disease	**Crohn's Disease**
Gender (M/F)	49–0.57	2.9–0.76
Symptoms onset age (yr)	20.8–40	15–29
Average age at diagnosis (yr)	24.7–35.7	29.5–31
Oral aphtous ulcers (%)	Approximately 100	< 10
Uveitis (%)	57–69	< 10
Skin lesions (%)	61–87	< 10
Arthritis (%)	30–57	2–24.7
Gastrointestinal involvement (%)		
Ileocecal area	50–94	40–83
Colon	10–15	32–50
Upper GI	1–3	4
Perianal	1–2	10–15
Intestinal complications (%)		
Perforation	12.7	8.7
Fistula	7.6	24.7
Stricture	7.2	38.3
Abscess	3.3	19.6
Endoscopic Morphology	Round-oval shape	Longitudinal ulcers with a cobblestone appearance
	Focal, solitary	segmental and diffuse distribution
	Volcano-shaped	
	Deep ulcers	
Mucosal Biopsy	Vasculitis	Granuloma
	Neutrophilic infiltration	Focal cryptitis
	Fibrinopurulent exudates	Nerve fiberhyperplasia
	Necrotic debris	Lymphoid aggregates

Table 5.
Distribution of similarities and differences in the differential diagnosis of Behçet's disease and Crohn's disease [2, 3, 7, 9, 10, 15, 57–59, 61, 67, 80].

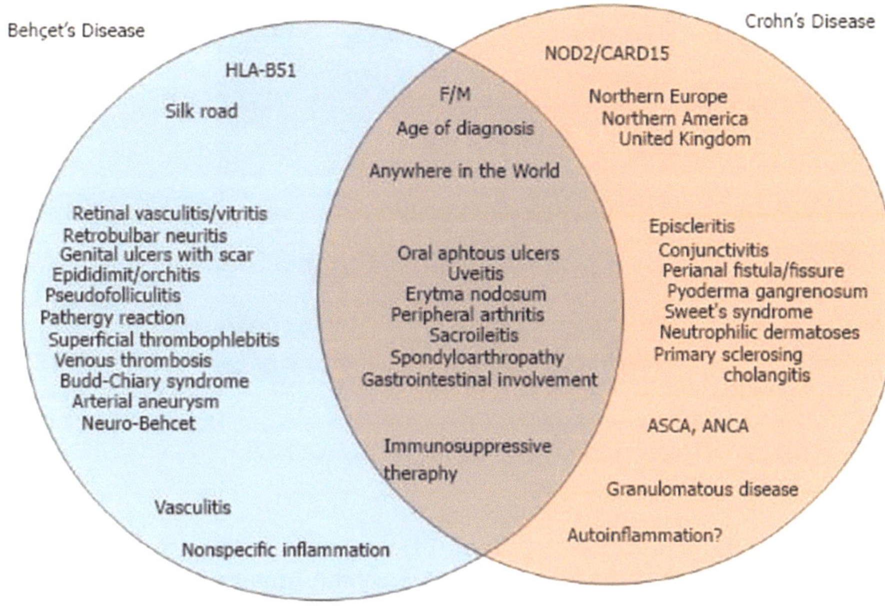

Figure 7.
Similar and different characteristics of Behçet's disease and Crohn's disease [60]. F: Female; M: Male; ASCA: Anti-Saccharomyces cerevisiae antibodies; ANCA: Anti-Saccharomyces cerevisiae antibodies; ANCA: Anti-neutrophil cytoplasmic antibodies.

6. Infectious colitis

Infectious colitis usually presents with sudden onset of symptoms (characterized as acute self-limited colitis). In developing countries, infectious colitis remains one of the most common causes of diarrhea that can mimic IBD. Colitis can be caused by bacterial and parasitic infections, ileitis can be the result of yersiniosis and salmonella infections, and ileocolonic ulcers can be seen with amebiasis. Symptoms of acute infectious colitis are sudden onset, early fever and diarrhea (more than 6 times a day), which can also be in the acute course (fulminant course) of CD. Extraintestinal symptoms and signs such as arthropathy, ophthalmic, and skin symptoms may also be present in acute self-limited colitis but are more common in CD. Stool examinations play an important role in confirming the diagnosis of infectious colitis. In such situations, endoscopy (sigmoidoscopy or total colonoscopy) with the collection of biopsies from the mucous membrane can be very informative.

Histological examination of the biopsy specimen in acute infectious colitis showed that the structure of the crypt was normal, the inflammation of the mucous membrane was predominantly acute; there is no increase in plasma cells or lymphoid aggregates at the base of the crypts. Histological examination of IBD biopsy samples, even in the early course, often reveals crypt deformity, basal plasmacytosis and basal lymphoid aggregates, as well as an increase in the number of cells in the lamina propria in the stages of acute and chronic inflammation [59]. But with the chronicity of the infectious process or with an inadequate choice of antimicrobial therapy, the histological picture begins to change with elements of the lesion

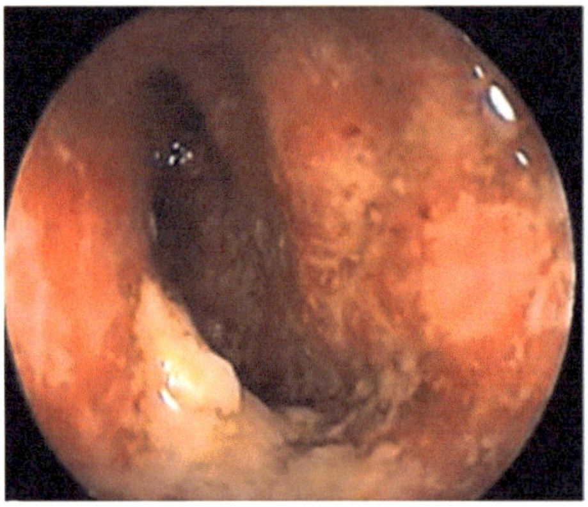

Figure 8.
Endoscopic image of chronic schistosomatous colitis (histologically verified) [5].

characteristic of the complicated course of IBD, in particular, the complicated course of Crohn's disease combined with an infectious agent. Chronic schistosomatous colitis may mimic a complicated course of Crohn's disease with concomitant infection (see **Figure 8**) [2, 5, 9, 60].

Enterohemorrhagic *E. coli*, which in most cases leads to the onset of ischemic colitis, can mimic an IBD-like lesion, and also occur with overlap syndromes in patients with CD, which makes diagnosis extremely difficult, since due to disturbances in the hemodynamic flow in patients with CD, it is quite ischemic bowel disease is common. The defeat of *E. coli* is characterized by the appearance of a neutrophilic cryptal abscess, more often localized in the upper half of the mucous membrane, and pronounced neutrophils in the lamina propria of the mucous membrane. Basal plasmacytosis, characteristic of IBD, is absent, the structure of the glands is normal, erosion and edema of the lamina propria of the mucous membrane are found (see **Figures 8** and **9**). The disease can stop on its own; its course correlates with what bacteria are found in the fecal masses. As the colitis subsides (which is quite common by the time a biopsy is taken), reactive changes in the epithelium are found in the biopsy specimens, but the shape of the crypts remains unchanged.

Intestinal amebiasis should be included in the differential diagnosis of CD and UC, not only in endemic countries. Some endoscopic and histological features may be useful for differential diagnosis, for example, at endoscopy in patients with amebiasis, discrete small ulcers 2 mm or less in diameter are most often detected in the caecum or rectosigmoid region. With regard to histology, amebic trophozoites are most often localized in necrotic material, mucin, proteinaceous material, and intestinal mucosa [61].

Necrotizing epithelioid granulomatous inflammation may occur in Yersinia pseudotuberculosis infections; in infection with Yersinia enterocolitica, accumulations of macrophages may be found. It is the formation of granulomas that creates difficulties for the morphologist in terms of determining their specificity for Crohn's disease. It is necessary to take into account the fact that with yersiniosis the granulomas are larger than with Crohn's disease. Morphological changes in pseudomembranous colitis are also similar to changes characteristic of CD. More Lamps et al. in 2000 pointed to the propensity of histioplasmosis of the gastrointestinal tract to cause changes similar to

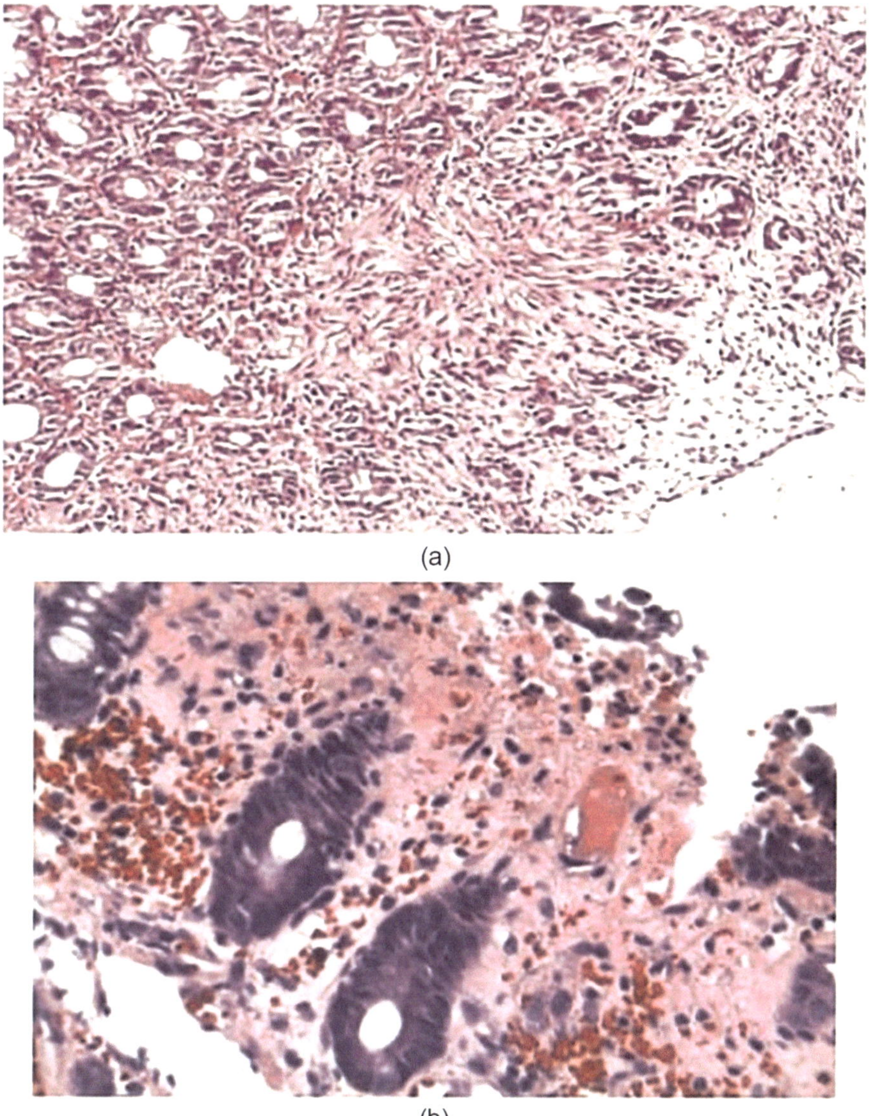

(a)

(b)

Figure 9.
*Morphological image of the biopsy material of the intestine (unpublished date from the archives of the authors (Musayev C.S.)). (a) Crohn's disease (biopsy fragment taken from the area of the mucous membrane of the caecum): formed granulomas in the lamina propria with accumulation of lymphocytes and histiocytes (stain: Hematoxylin and Eosin; magnification: x200). (b) infectious colitis (*E. Coli O157:H7*): diffuse hemorrhages, swelling, erosion, lymphocytic and neutrophilic infiltration of the colon mucosa (stain: Hematoxylin and Eosin; magnification: x200).*

those in CD. These two pathologies are quite often manifested by common symptoms: fever, weakness, gastrointestinal bleeding, diarrhea, nausea, vomiting, ulcers and cracks, perforation, and due to the presence of granulomas and inflammatory changes that capture the entire thickness of the intestinal wall, they are quite often mistaken for Crohn's disease.

Lymphogranuloma venereum is a disease caused by three unique strains of Chlamydia trachomatis and characterized by small, often asymptomatic skin lesions accompanied by localized enlargement of the lymph nodes in the groin or pelvis. If infection occurred due to anal sex, then it can manifest itself in the form of severe proctitis. Venereal lymphogranuloma occurs in three stages.

Stage 1 begins after an incubation period of approximately 3 days with a small skin lesion at the site of contact. This can cause cracks (ulceration) to appear on the top layer of the skin, but they heal so quickly that it may go unnoticed.

Stage 2 usually begins in men after about 2 to 4 weeks, with enlargement of the inguinal lymph nodes on one or both sides and the formation of large, painful, sometimes fluctuating masses (buboes). The buboes penetrate deeper tissues and make the top layer of the skin inflamed, sometimes accompanied by fever and malaise. In women, low back or pelvic pain is common; the initial lesions may be on the cervix or upper part of the vagina, leading to enlargement and deeper inflammation of the perirectal and pelvic lymph nodes. Multiple drainage fistulas may appear, through which pus or blood comes out.

In stage 3, lesions heal with scarring, but fistula cavities may remain or reappear. The persistent inflammation from an untreated infection clogs the lymphatic vessels, causing skin sores and swelling.

People who practice anal sex in a passive role at the 1st stage may suffer from severe proctitis or proctocolitis with bloody-purulent rectal discharge. In the chronic stages, colitis mimicking Crohn's disease can cause tenesmus and strictures in the rectum or pain due to inflamed inguinal lymph nodes. Proctoscopy may reveal diffuse inflammation, polyps and masses, or mucopurulent exudate, symptoms that closely resemble inflammatory bowel disease.

A similar clinical, endoscopic and morphological picture with rectal CD is characteristic of sexually transmitted infections (see **Table 6**).

Infections not only mimic CD, but can also worsen the course and outcome of CD treatment. Thorough screening for infections is always necessary before making a diagnosis of IBD and initiating immunosuppressive treatment in these patients.

7. Diseases of the vascular system mimicking IBD

Various diseases based on damage to the vascular system can mimic IBD.

Systemic vasculitis is a heterogeneous group of diseases and is classified depending on the type and size of vessels involved in the pathological process, which, in turn, determines the area and type of ischemic damage [62, 63]. Depending on the type of vasculitis, intestinal involvement ranges from widespread intestinal infarcts in large vessel vasculitis to focal, segmental ischemia and ulceration due to intramural artery involvement in small vessel vasculitis [62, 64]. Clinically, the intestinal manifestations of vasculitis range from mild abdominal pain to serious and potentially life-threatening complications such as peritonitis and intestinal perforation. The frequency and type of these intestinal manifestations depends on the type of systemic vasculitis. The most common intestinal manifestations of systemic vasculitis are given in **Table** 7.

Clinical symptoms of intestinal damage may be detected at the initial manifestation of the disease or occur during a relapse; may be the only manifestation of the disease.

Diagnosis of intestinal involvement within systemic vasculitis can be quite challenging for the clinician. Patients with GI involvement associated with systemic vasculitis usually present with a range of nonspecific complaints: fever, abdominal pain, nausea, vomiting, diarrhea, and gastrointestinal bleeding. For diagnosis, the most informative are instrumental research methods. So, for example, catheter angiography

Gonorrheal proctitis	*Clinically:* Pain in the rectum and anus, purulent, mucous, spotting, tenesmus, imperative urge to defecate are possible *Endoscopically:* picture of non-specific ulcerative lesions *Histologically:* corresponds to acute nonspecific proctitis
Chlamydial proctitis	*Clinically:* Pain in the rectum and anus, purulent, mucous, spotting, tenesmus, imperative urge to defecate are possible *Endoscopically:* ulcer picture *Histologically:* it resembles Crohn's disease (the predominance of lymphohistiocytic and plasmacytic infiltration of the submucosa, muscular and serous membranes with hyperplasia of the elements of the submucosal and muscular-intestinal plexuses is characteristic, excessive thickening and fibrosis of the intestinal wall can be detected, spreading only within the rectum, specific in surface biopsy changes may not be
Proctitis syphilis	*Clinically:* Pain in the rectum and anus, purulent, mucous, spotting, tenesmus, imperative urge to defecate are possible *Endoscopically:* granularity, slight vulnerability, hyperemia, thickening or ulceration of the mucous membrane *Histologically:* neutrophilic cryptitis with ulceration, granulation tissue and marked lymphoplasmacytic infiltration of the adjacent mucosa and submucosa, immature granulomas may be found

Table 6.
Clinical, endoscopic and histological signs of infectious proctitis caused by pathogens of sexually transmitted infections.

Vasculitis	Intestinal manifestations and their frequency
Vasculitis of large vessels	
Arteritis Takayasu (non-specific aortoarteritis)	Vascular murmurs (14%) [65]; diffuse ischemia of the gastrointestinal tract (4%) [65]; stenotic or occlusive lesions in the abdominal aorta and/or superior mesenteric arteries (25%) [66].
Giant cell arteritis	Mesenteric ischemia [67].
Medium vessel vasculitis	
Polyarteritis nodosa	Abdominal pain (up to 95%) [68, 69]; intestinal ulcers (5–6%) [68, 69]; narrowed cone-shaped and/or saccular arteries, fusiform microaneurysms in the mesenteric arteries (85%) [70]; occlusions and stenosis of the superior mesenteric arteries, infarcts and thickening of the intestinal wall [71].
Kawasaki disease	paralytic ileus, appendicular vasculitis and hemorrhagic duodenitis (5–20%) [72, 73].
Vasculitis of small vessels	
ANCA-associated vasculitis	Mucosal ulcers, intestinal infarction, ischemia, perforation or occlusion (20–50%) [68]; MPA: ischemic colon ulcers, peritonitis and intestinal perforation [68, 74]; GPA and EGPA: granulomatous ulceration of the colon (may mimic IBD) [68].

Vasculitis	Intestinal manifestations and their frequency
IgA vasculitis (Schonlein-Henoch purpura)	Mucous purpura (20–50%) with gastrointestinal bleeding (18–52%) [75, 76]; swelling of the intestinal mucosa, infarction, diffuse hyperemia of the mucous membrane, hemorrhagic erosions, perforation or invagination (3–5%) [75, 76].
Cryoglobulinemic vasculitis	Intestinal ischemia (80%) [68, 77].
Behçet's disease	Ileocecal ulcers [47]

Notes: ANCA, anti-neutrophil cytoplasmic antibodies; IBD, inflammatory bowel disease; MPA, microscopic polyangiitis; EGPA, eosinophilic granulomotosis with polyangiitis; GPA - granulomatosis with polyangiities.

Table 7.
Intestinal manifestations of systemic vasculitis.

of blood vessels is the "gold standard" for diagnosis in case of suspected damage to the mesenteric vessels. Computed tomography and magnetic resonance angiography can also be useful for diagnosing gastrointestinal vascular lesions in vasculitis [78].

Endoscopic examination in patients with suspected bowel involvement as part of systemic vasculitis is a less informative diagnostic method. Due to the increased risk of perforation in ischemic conditions inherent in systemic vasculitis, endoscopy should be performed with extreme caution. Video capsule endoscopy can be useful for visualizing lesions of the small intestine, areas of which are not accessible to conventional endoscopy, but the lack of a biopsy significantly reduces the information content of the method [62, 64]. Colonoscopic symptoms in the acute period often include edematous friable mucosa, erythema, and disseminated pale areas. More severe disease is characterized by mucosal cyanosis, diffuse hemorrhagic erosions, and/or linear ulceration [62, 64]. In the chronic phase of intestinal ischemia, mucosal atrophy and areas of granulation tissue can be detected.

Biopsies taken from affected areas may show nonspecific changes such as hemorrhage, ruptured crypts, capillary thrombosis, tissue granulation with abscesses, and pseudopolyps [62, 64]. Biopsy material taken from the area of post-ischemic stricture is characterized by extensive transmural fibrosis and mucosal atrophy.

At the moment, there is no single highly informative diagnostic laboratory test for vasculitis. Basic laboratory tests are most often used to determine the extent of organ damage and the extent of organ involvement. More specific serological tests, including antineutrophil cytoplasmic antibodies (ANCA), can also additionally help in the diagnosis of systemic vasculitis, but given the fact that in 60–70% of patients with UC, the ANCA test may be positive, then again the question differential diagnosis becomes debatable. The scientific literature presents an association of Takayasu's arteritis with inflammatory bowel disease, suggesting a possible link between the two entities. In a North American cohort of 160 patients with Takayasu's arteritis, 8 patients (5%) were diagnosed with IBD compared with a 0.2% prevalence of Crohn's disease in the general population [79]. There is evidence of a genetic overlap between Takayasu's arteritis and ulcerative colitis: the presence of HLA B52:01 as a common genetic determinant [80]. The diagnosis of IBD usually precedes the development of Takayasu's arteritis (on average by 4 years) [62, 79].

It should be noted that the coexistence of these two diseases does not imply a worse prognosis for either IBD or Takayasu's arteritis.

Granulomatosis with polyangiitis (GPA) is the most common primary systemic vasculitis. This is an autoimmune granulomatous inflammation of the walls of blood vessels, involving small and medium-sized blood vessels: capillaries, venules, arterioles, and arteries, with involvement of the upper respiratory tract, eyes, kidneys, lungs, and other organs [41, 62]. GPA is commonly associated with PR3-ANCA. Gastrointestinal symptoms occur in 5–11% of patients with GPA [81, 82]. Autopsy studies revealed histopathological evidence of gastrointestinal vasculitis in 24% of GPA cases. Any part of the gastrointestinal tract can be involved in the pathological process, but the most common are lesions of the small and large intestine. Symptoms range from transient abdominal pain and ulcers (oral, esophageal, and peptic) to bloody diarrhea and intestinal perforation [83]. Gastrointestinal imaging findings are generally nonspecific, ranging from multifocal or diffuse bowel wall thickening to mesenteric vascular stasis and ascites [70].

Endoscopy may reveal ulceration, sometimes described as granulomatous and ischemic changes. Compared with Crohn's disease, the ulcers seen in GPA are more often shallow and transversely oriented, but making a differential diagnosis is difficult, as cases of concomitant Crohn's disease (or ulcerative colitis) in GPA (or other autoimmune-associated vasculitis) have been described [79, 83, 84]. Standard endoscopic biopsy of colon ulcers has a low sensitivity ($\sim$ 30–40%), but if the material is taken from deep layers, the specificity of the study increases. However, taking deep biopsies has a high risk of perforation in patients with vasculitis [62, 64].

In the scientific literature, there are also indications of the frequent coexistence of EGPA and IBD [79].

The main clinical manifestations in most patients with eosinophilic granulomatosis with polyangiitis (EGPA) are late-onset asthma, eosinophilia, cutaneous vasculitis (purpura), and/or multifocal mononeuritis. Serum MPO-ANCA is found in 30–40% of patients with EGPA. Cardiac involvement, more common in ANCA-negative patients, is a major risk factor for mortality [62, 63, 85]. In the study by Tsurikisawa et al. (2015) studied the pathology of the gastrointestinal tract and the role of T-helpers 17(Th17) in the pathogenesis of gastrointestinal manifestations in patients with EGPA. They had elevated levels of Th17 and serum intercellular adhesion molecule 1 (ICAM-1), colonic eosinophilia, and submucosal edema, which decreased in remission [86]. Similar changes are observed in IBD. Intestinal symptoms occur in 30–50% of patients with EGPA and are nonspecific and include abdominal pain (91%), diarrhea (45%), melena or hematochezia (19–36%), nausea and vomiting (18%), and acute stomach (6–36%).

Mesenteric artery vasculitis is the most common explanation for these manifestations and can lead to intestinal infarction and perforation, especially in the small intestine. Infiltration of the intestinal mucosa by eosinophils can also cause pain, dysmotility, obstructive symptoms, and diarrhea with the development of eosinophilic colitis. Granulomatous and eosinophilic mucosal ulcers have been described as potential sources of bleeding in the jejunum and/or, less commonly, the colon [68, 87].

8. Conclusion

As can be seen from the above material, the diagnosis of IBD continues to be a serious problem. We have considered only the most common pathologies that mimic the clinical picture of IBD. At the same time, one should not forget about drug-induced damage to the intestines (sodium phosphate, non-steroidal anti-inflammatory drugs, proton pump inhibitors, mycophenolate mofetil, chemotherapy drugs for oncological diseases, etc.).

For this reason, only a detailed collection of the patient's history and a precisely adjusted examination plan can provide enough material to establish the correct diagnosis.

Lack of physician awareness of immune-inflammatory diseases, iatrogenesis, opportunistic infections, and, in certain cases, limited availability of some expensive diagnostic methods, as well as the lack of a state program for the prevention, diagnosis, treatment and rehabilitation of IBD, can lead to diagnostic errors. The incidence of IBD has increased over the past two decades and is expected to continue to rise in the next decade. To date, there are several global recommendations for the diagnosis and treatment of IBD in the world, which help to make the diagnosis accurate and the treatment standardized. Given the high prevalence of infectious enteritis/colitis, tuberculosis, Behçet's disease, and systemic vasculitis, careful differentiation is always necessary before a diagnosis of IBD is made.

The realities of the status quo underscore the need for innovation in the healthcare system:

1. Based on the data obtained after conducting population studies, it is necessary to develop a National Health Care Program by creating an adapted National Guideline and the Center for the Study of IBD;

2. Improve the program of continuing medical education, incl. as part of a multidisciplinary approach for doctors of related specialties.

3. These measures will reduce the time to establish an accurate diagnosis, and due to the involvement of specialists in related pathologies in conditions overlapping with IBD, timely prescribe adequate therapy and achieve a decrease in disability and death rates in this category of patients.

Conflict of interest

The authors declare no conflict of interest.

Author details

Gulustan H. Babayeva[1*], Gunay V. Asadova[1,2], Jamal S. Musayev[3], Umud R. Mahmudov[4], Farid V. Quliyev[2] and Aychin I. Hasanova[1]

1 Department of Therapy, Azerbaijan State Advanced Training Institute for Doctors Named After A.Alıyev, Baku, Azerbaijan

2 Department of Invasive Diagnostic and Treatment, National Centre of Oncology, Baku, Azerbaijan

3 Baku Pathology Center, Baku, Azerbaijan

4 Department of Gastroenterology and Endoscopy, Modern Hospital, Baku, Azerbaijan

*Address all correspondence to: ghbabayeva@gmail.com

References

[1] Ananthakrishnan AN, Kaplan GG, Ng SC. Changing global epidemiology of inflammatory bowel diseases: Sustaining health care delivery into the 21st century. Clinical Gastroenterology and Hepatology. 2020; **18**(6):1252-1260. DOI: 10.1016/j.cgh.2020.01.028

[2] Li Y, Qian J-M. The challenge of inflammatory bowel disease diagnosis in Asia. Inflamm Intest Dis. 2016;**1**:159-164. DOI: 10.1159/000448384

[3] Ng SC, Hirai HW, Tsoi KF, et al. Systematic review with meta-analysis: Accuracy of interferon-gamma releasing assay and anti-Saccharomyces cerevisiae antibody in differentiating intestinal tuberculosis from Crohn's disease in Asians. Journal of Gastroenterology and Hepatology. 2014;**29**:1664-1670

[4] Lee YJ, Yang SK, Byeon JS, Myung SJ, et al. Analysis of colonoscopic findings in the differential diagnosis between intestinal tuberculosis and Crohn's disease. Endoscopy. 2006;**38**: 592-597

[5] Li X, Liu X, Zou Y, Ouyang C, Wu X, et al. Predictors of clinical and endoscopic findings in differentiating Crohn's disease from intestinal tuberculosis. Digestive Diseases and Sciences. 2011;**56**:188-196

[6] Pattanayak S, Behuria S. Is abdominal tuberculosis a surgical problem? Annals of the Royal College of Surgeons of England. 2015;**97**(6):414-419

[7] Kumarasinghe MP, Quek TP, Chau CY, Mustapha NR, et al. Endoscopic biopsy features and diagnostic challenges of adult Crohn's disease at initial presentation. Pathology. 2010;**42**:131-137

[8] Chee CB, Barkham TM, KhinMar KW, et al. Quantitative T-cell interferon-gamma responses to Mycobacterium tuberculosis-specific antigens in active and latent tuberculosis. European Journal of Clinical Microbiology & Infectious Diseases. 2009;**28**:667-670

[9] Li Y, Zhang LF, Liu XQ, et al. The role of in vitro interferonγ-release assay in differentiating intestinal tuberculosis from Crohn's disease in China. Journal of Crohn's & Colitis. 2012;**6**:317-323

[10] Gan HT, Chen YQ, Ouyang Q, Bu H, Yang XY. Differentiation between intestinal tuberculosis and Crohn's disease in endoscopic biopsy specimens by polymerase chain reaction. The American Journal of Gastroenterology. 2002;**97**:1446-1451

[11] Pulimood AB, Peter S, Rook GWA, Donoghue HD. In situ PCR for mycobacterium tuberculosis in endoscopic mucosal biopsy specimens of intestinal tuberculosis and Crohn disease. American Journal of Clinical Pathology. 2008;**129**:846-851

[12] Ramadass B, Chittaranjan S, Subramanian V, Ramakrishna BS. Fecal polymerase chain reaction for Mycobacterium tuberculosis IS6110 to distinguish Crohn's disease from intestinal tuberculosis. Indian Journal of Gastroenterology. 2010;**29**:152-156

[13] Park YH, Chung WS, Lim JS, et al. Diagnostic role of computed tomographic enterography differentiating Crohn disease from intestinal tuberculosis. Journal of Computer Assisted Tomography. 2013; **37**:834-839

[14] Mao R, Liao WD, He Y, Ouyang CH, et al. Computed tomographic enterography adds value to colonoscopy in differentiating Crohn's disease from intestinal tuberculosis: A potential diagnostic algorithm. Endoscopy. 2015; **47**:322-329

[15] Tahiri M, Goh KL, Abbas Z, Epstein D, Min-Hu C, Mulder C, et al. Global Guidelines Digestive Tract Tuberculosis. © World Gastroentero-logy Organisation Global Guidelines; 2021

[16] Sood A, Midha V, Singh A. Differential diagnosis of Crohn's disease versus ileal tuberculosis. Current Gastroenterology Reports. 2014;**16**(11): 418

[17] Almadi MA, Ghosh S, Aljebreen AM. Differentiating intestinal tuberculosis from Crohn's disease: A diagnostic challenge. The American Journal of Gastroenterology. 2009; **104**(4):1003

[18] He Y, Zhu Z, Chen Y, Chen F, Wang Y, Ouyang C, et al. Development and validation of a novel diagnostic nomogram to differentiate between intestinal tuberculosis and Crohn's disease: A 6- year prospective multicenter study. The American Journal of Gastroenterology. 2019;**114**(3): 490-499

[19] Triantafillidis JK, Thomaidis T, Papalois A. Terminal ileitis due to yersinia infection: An underdiagnosed situation. BioMed Research International. 2020;**2020**:1240626. DOI: 10.1155/2020/1240626

[20] Bockemühl J, Roggentin P. Intestinal yersiniosis. Clinical importance, epidemiology, diagnosis, and prevention. Bundesgesundheitsblatt, Gesundheitsforschung, Gesundheitsschutz. 2004;**47**(7):685-691. DOI: 10.1007/s00103-004-0865-9

[21] Le Guern AS, Martin L, Savin C, Carniel E. Yersiniosis in France: Overview and potential sources of infection. International Journal of Infectious Diseases. 2016;**46**:1-7. DOI: 10.1016/j.ijid.2016.03.008

[22] Chlebicz A, Śliżewska K. Campylobacteriosis, Salmonellosis, Yersiniosis, and Listeriosis as zoonotic foodborne diseases: A review. International Journal of Environmental Research and Public Health. 2018;**15**(5): 863. DOI: 10.3390/ijerph15050863

[23] Zadernowska A, Chajęcka-Wierzchowska W, Ogryzek MP. Growth potential of Yersinia enterocolitica in blue cheese and in blue cheese with probiotic–Lactobacillus acidophilus LA-5®. Journal of Food Science and Technology. 2015;**52**(11): 7540-7544. DOI: 10.1007/s13197-015-1873-5

[24] Garrido E, Sanromán AL, Rodríguez-Gandía MA, et al. Optimized protocol for diagnosis of acute ileitis. Clinical Gastroenterology and Hepatology. 2009;**7**(11):1183-1188. DOI: 10.1016/j.cgh.2009.07.014

[25] Le Baut G, O'Brien C, Pavli P, et al. Prevalence of Yersinia species in the ileum of Crohn's disease patients and controls. Frontiers in Cellular and Infection Microbiology. 2018;**8** (336):1-9. DOI: 10.3389/fcimb.2018. 00336

[26] Tomaso H, Mooseder G, Dahouk SA, et al. Seroprevalence of anti-Yersinia antibodies in healthy Austrians. European Journal of Epidemiology. 2006;**21**(1):77-81. DOI: 10.1007/ s10654-005-5047-z

[27] Knösel T, Schewe C, Petersen N, Dietel M, Petersen I. Prevalence of infectious pathogens in Crohn's disease. Pathology - Research and Practice. 2009; **205**(4):223-230. DOI: 10.1016/j.prp.2008.04.018

[28] Jess T, Jess P. Acute terminal ileitis, yersiniosis, and Crohn's disease: A long-term follow-up study of the relationships. European Journal of Internal Medicine. 2001;**12**(2):98-100. DOI: 10.1016/S0953-6205(01)00122-4

[29] Rosner BM, Stark K, Werber D. Epidemiology of reported Yersinia enterocolitica infections in Germany, 2001-2008. BMC Public Health. 2010;**10**: 337, 1-8. DOI: 10.1186/1471-2458-10-337

[30] Vantrappen G, Ponette E, Geboes K, Bertrand P. Yersinia enteritis and enterocolitis: Gastroenterological aspects. Gastroenterology. 1977;**72**(2):220-227. DOI: 10.1016/S0016-5085(77)80076-0

[31] Jones MW, Godana I, Deppen JG. StatPearls. In: Pseudoappendicitis. Treasure Island, FL, USA: Stat Pearls Publishing; 2020 Available from: https://www.ncbi.nlm.nih.gov/books/NBK499946/

[32] Tse CS, Deepak P, Smyrk TC, Raffals LE. Isolated acute terminal ileitis without preexisting inflammatory bowel disease rarely progresses to Crohn's disease. Digestive Diseases and Sciences. 2017;**62**(12):3557-3562. DOI: 10.1007/s10620-017-4803-8

[33] Laji N, Bowyer R, Jeyaratnam D, Zuckerman M. Another mistaken case of appendicitis. Hindawi BioMed Research International. **2020**:10. Article ID 1240626. DOI: 10.1155/2020/1240626

[34] Mert M, Kocabay G, Ozülker T, et al. Liver abscess due to Yersinia bacteremia in a well-controlled type I diabetic patient. Endokrynologia Polska. 2011; **62**(4):357-360

[35] Kaasch AJ, Dinter J, Goeser T, Plum G, Seifert H. Yersinia pseudotuberculosis bloodstream infection and septic arthritis: Case report and review of the literature. Infection. 2012;**40**(2):185-190. DOI: 10.1007/s15010-011-0160-2

[36] Safa G, Loppin M, Tisseau L, Lamoril J. Cutaneous aseptic neutrophilic abscesses and Yersinia enterocolitica infection in a case subsequently diagnosed as Crohn's disease. Dermatology. 2008;**217**(4): 340-342. DOI: 10.1159/000155646

[37] Zippi M, Colaiacomo MC, Marcheggiano A, et al. Mesenteric adenitis caused by Yersinia pseudotubercolosis in a patient subsequently diagnosed with Crohn's disease of the terminal ileum. World Journal of Gastroenterology. 2006; **12**(24):3933-3935. DOI: 10.3748/wjg.v12.i24.3933

[38] Homewood R, Gibbons CP, Richards D, Lewis A, Duane PD, Griffiths AP. Ileitis due to Yersinia pseudotuberculosis in Crohn's disease. Journal of Infection. 2003;**47**(4):328-332. DOI: 10.1016/S0163-4453(03)00064-1

[39] Naddei R, Martinelli M, Strisciuglio C, et al. Yersinia enterocolitica ileitis mimicking pediatric Crohn's disease. Inflammatory Bowel Diseases. 2017;**23**(4):E15-E16. DOI: 10.1097/MIB.0000000000001052

[40] Greco L, Marino F, Gentile A, Catalano G, Angilletta D. Yersinia enterocolitica ileocolitis in beta-thalassemic patients. Colorectal Disease. 2006;**8**(6):525. DOI: 10.1111/j.1463-1318.2006.01010.x

[41] Warner B, Jayasooriya N, Sanderson J, Anderson S, Irving P. Yersinia - A rarer cause of terminal ileitis. Archives of Case Reports in Clinical Medicine. 2016;**2**(3): 123, 4 pages. DOI: 10.19104/crcm.2016.123

[42] Saebo A, Vik E, Lange OJ, Matuszkiewicz L. Inflammatory bowel disease associated with Yersinia enterocolitica O:3 infection. European Journal of Internal Medicine. 2005;**16**(3): 176-182. DOI: 10.1016/j.ejim.2004.11.008

[43] Matsumoto T, Iida M, Matsui T, et al. Endoscopic findings in Yersinia enterocolitica enterocolitis. Gastrointestinal Endoscopy. 1990;**36**(6):583-587. DOI: 10.1016/S0016-5107(90)71169-8

[44] El-Maraghi NR, Mair NS. The histopathology of enteric infection with Yersinia pseudotuberculosis. American Journal of Clinical Pathology. 1979;**71**(6): 631-639

[45] Montgomery EA, Popek EJ. Intussusception, adenovirus, and children: A brief reaffirmation. Human Pathology. 1994;**25**:169-174

[46] Montgomery EA et al. Biopsy interpretation of gastrointestinal tract mucosa. In: Non-Neoplastic. Vol. 1. Lippinncton: Williams& Wilkins; 2012

[47] Skef W, Hamilton MJ, Arayssi T. Gastrointestinal Behçet's disease: A review. World Journal of Gastroenterology. 2015;**21**(13): 3801-3812. DOI: 10.3748/wjg.v21.i13.3801

[48] Kim DH, Cheon JH. Intestinal Behçet's disease: A true inflammatory bowel disease or merely an intestinal complication of systemic vasculitis? Yonsei Medical Journal. 2016;**57**(1): 22-32. DOI: 10.3349/ymj.2016.57.1.22

[49] Criteria for diagnosis of Behçet's disease. International study group for Behçet's disease. Lancet. 1990;**335**:1078

[50] Bayraktar Y, Ozaslan E, Van Thiel DH. Gastrointestinal manifestations of Behçet's disease. Journal of Clinical Gastroenterology. 2000;**30**:144-154

[51] Watanabe K, Tanida S, Inoue N, Kunisaki R, Kobayashi K, et al. Evidence-based diagnosis and clinical practice guidelines for intestinal Behçet's disease 2020 edited by intractable diseases, the health and labour sciences research grants. Journal of Gastroenterology. 2020;**55**:679-700

[52] Hisamatsu T, Ueno F, Matsumoto T, et al. The 2nd edition of consensus statements for the diagnosis and management of intestinal Behcet's disease: Indication of anti-TNFalpha monoclonal antibodies. Journal of Gastroenterology. 2014;**49**:156-162

[53] Suzuki Kurokawa M, Suzuki N. Behcet's disease. Clinical and Experimental Medicine. 2004;**4**:10-20

[54] Vaiopoulos AG, Sfikakis PP, Kanakis MA, et al. Gastrointestinal manifestations of Behçet's disease: Advances in evaluation and management. Clinical and Experimental Rheumatology. 2014;**32**(4Suppl 84): S140-S148

[55] Moon CM, Cheon JH, Shin JK, et al. Prediction of free bowel perforation in patients with intestinal Behçet's disease using clinical and colonoscopic findings. Digestive Diseases and Sciences. 2010;**55**: 2904-2911

[56] Li J, Li P, Bai J, Lyu H, et al. Discriminating potential of extraintestinal systemic manifestations

and colonoscopic features in Chinese patients with intestinal Behçet's disease and Crohn's disease. Chinese Medical Journal. 2015;**128**:233-238

[57] Cheon JH, Kim ES, Shin SJ, Kim TI, et al. Development and validation of novel diagnostic criteria for intestinal Behçet's disease in Korean patients with ileocolonic ulcers. The American Journal of Gastroenterology. 2009;**104**: 2492-2499

[58] Yazısız V. Similarities and differences between Behçet's disease and Crohn's disease. World J Gastrointest Pathophysiol. 2014;**5**(3):228-238. DOI: 10.4291/wjgp.v5.i3.228

[59] Surawicz CM, Haggitt RC, Hussemann M, McFarland LV. Mucosal biopsy diagnosis of colitis: acute self-limited colitis and acute idiopathic inflammatory bowel disease. Gastroenterology. 1994;**107**: 755-763

[60] Cao J, Liu WJ, Xu XY, Zou XP. Endoscopic findings and clinicopathologic characteristics of colonic schistosomiasis: A report of 46 cases. World Journal of Gastroenterology. 2010;**16**:723-727

[61] Singh R, Balekuduru A, Simon EG, et all. The differentiation of amebic colitis from inflammatory bowel disease on endoscopic mucosal biopsies. Indian Journal of Pathology & Microbiology. 2015;**58**:427-432

[62] Golovach Y, Yehudina Ye.D. Gastrointestinal manifestations of systemic vasculitis: a spectrum of clinical manifestations, diagnosis and treatment. Gastroenterologia. 2019;**53**(4):291-304. DOI: 10.22141/2308-2097.53.3.2019. 182405

[63] Jennette JC, Falk RJ, Bacon PA, et al. 2012 revised International Chapel Hill Consensus Conference Nomenclature of Vasculitides. Arthritis and Rheumatism 2013;**65**(1):1-11. DOI: 10.1002/art.37715.

[64] Hatemi I, Hatemi G, Çelik AF. Systemic vasculitis and the gut. Current Opinion in Rheumatology. 2017;**29**(1): 33-38. DOI: 10.1097/ BOR.000000000 0000344

[65] Schmidt J, Kermani TA, Bacani AK, et al. Diagnostic features, treatment, and outcomes of Takayasu arteritis in a US cohort of 126 patients. Mayo Clinic Proceedings. 2013;**88**(8):822-830. DOI: 10.1016/j.mayocp.2013.04.025

[66] Reddi A, Chetty R. Primary aorto-esophageal fistula due to Takayasu's aortitis. Cardiovascular Pathology. 2003; **12**(2):112-114

[67] Scola CJ, Li C, Upchurch KS. Mesenteric involvement in giant cell arteritis. An underrecognized complication? Analysis of a case series with clinicoanatomic correlation. Medicine (Baltimore). 2008; **87**(1):45-51. DOI: 10.1097/MD.0b013 e3181646118

[68] Pagnoux C, Mahr A, Cohen P, Guillevin L. Presentation and outcome of gastrointestinal involvement in systemic necrotizing vasculitides: analysis of 62 patients with polyarteritis nodosa, microscopic polyangiitis, Wegener granulomatosis, Churg–Strauss syndrome, or rheumatoid arthritis-associated vasculitis. Medicine (Baltimore). 2005;**84**(2):115-128. DOI: 10.1097/01.md. 0000158825. 87055.0b

[69] Pagnoux C, Seror R, Henegar C, et al. Clinical features and outcomes in 348 patients with polyarteritis nodosa: a systematic retrospective study of

patients diagnosed between 1963 and 2005 and entered into the French vasculitis study group database. Arthritis and Rheumatism. 2010;**62**(2):616-626. DOI: 10.1002/art.27240

[70] Ha HK, Lee SH, Rha SE, et al. Radiologic features of vasculitis involving the gastrointestinal tract. Radiographics. 2000;**20**(3):779-794. DOI: 10.1148/radiographics.20.3.g00mc02779

[71] Singhal M, Gupta P, Sharma A, Lal A, Rathi M, Khandelwal N. Role of multidetector abdominal CT in the evaluation of abnormalities in polyarteritis nodosa. Clinical Radiology. 2016;**71**(3):222-227. DOI: 10.1016/j.crad.2015.11.004

[72] Zulian F, Falcini F, Zancan L, et al. Acute surgical abdomen as presenting manifestation of Kawasaki disease. The Journal of Pediatrics. 2003; **142**(6):731-735. DOI: 10.1067/mpd.2003.232

[73] Singh R, Ward C, Walton M, Persad R. Atypical Kawasaki disease and gastrointestinal manifestations. Paediatrics & Child Health. 2007; **12**(3):235-237. DOI: 10.1093/pch/12.3.235

[74] Schirmer JH, Wright MN, Vonthein R, et al. Clinical presentation and long-term outcome of 144 patients with microscopic polyangiitis in a monocentric German cohort. Rheumatology (Oxford, England). 2016; **55**(1):71-79. DOI: 10.1093/rheumatology/kev286

[75] Chernyshova O, Gerasymenko V, Yegudina E, Syniachenko O, Ermolaeva M. The evolution of juvenile Schönlein-Henoch purpura. Child's Health. 2021;7 (75):85-89. DOI: 10.22141/2224-0551.7.75.2016.86730

[76] Ebert EC. Gastrointestinal manifestations of Henoch– Schönlein purpura. Digestive Diseases and Sciences. 2008;**53**(8):2011-2019. DOI: 10.1007/s10620-007-0147-0

[77] Cacoub P, Comarmond C, Domont F, Savey L, Saadoun D. Cryoglobulinemia vasculitis. The American Journal of Medicine. 2015 Sep; **128**(9):950-955. DOI: 10.1016/j.amjmed.2015.02.017

[78] Stone JR, Wilkins LR. Acute mesenteric ischemia. Techniques in Vascular and Interventional Radiology. 2015;**18**(1):24-30. DOI: 10.1053/j.tvir.2014.12.004

[79] Sy A, Khalidi N, Dehghan N, et al. Vasculitis in patients with inflammatory bowel diseases: A study of 32 patients and systematic review of the literature. Seminars in Arthritis and Rheumatism. 2016;**45**(4):475-482. DOI: 10.1016/j.semarthrit.2015.07.006

[80] Terao C, Matsumura T, Yoshifuji H, et al. Takayasu arteritis and ulcerative colitis: High rate of co-occurrence ratio and genetic overlap. Arthritis & Rhematology. 2015;**67**(8):2226-2232. DOI: 10.1002/ art.39157

[81] Nay J, Menias CO, Mellnick VM, Balfe DM. Gastrointestinal manifestations of systemic disease: a multimodality review. Abdominal Imaging. 2015;**40**(6):1926-1943. DOI: 10.1007/s00261-014-0334-3

[82] Akbulut S. Multiple ileal perforations in a patient with Wegener's granulomatosis: A case report and literature review. Journal of Gastrointestinal Surgery. 2012;**16**(4): 857-862. DOI: 10.1007/s11605-011-1735-z

[83] Humbert S, Guilpain P, Puéchal X, et al. Inflammatory bowel diseases in

anti-neutrophil cytoplasmic antibody-associated vasculitides: 11 retrospective cases from the French vasculitis study group. Rheumatology (Oxford, England). 2015;**54**(11):1970-1975. DOI: 10.1093/rheumatology/kev199

[84] Groh M, Pagnoux C, Baldini C, et al. Eosinophilic granulomatosis with polyangiitis (Churg–Strauss) (EGPA) consensus task force recommendations for evaluation and management. European Journal of Internal Medicine. 2015;**26**(7):545-553. DOI: 10.1016/j.ejim.2015.04.022

[85] Comarmond C, Pagnoux C, Khellaf M, et al. Eosinophilic granulomatosis with polyangiitis (Churg–Strauss): Clinical characteristics and long-term followup of the 383 patients enrolled in the French vasculitis study group cohort. Arthritis and Rheumatism. 2013;**65**(1):270-281. DOI: 10.1002/art.37721

[86] Tsurikisawa N, Oshikata C, Tsuburai T, et al. Th17 cells reflect colon submucosal pathologic changes in active eosinophilic granulomatosis with polyangiitis. BMC Immunology. 2015; **29**(16):75. DOI: 10.1186/s12865-015-0138-4

[87] Moosig F, Bremer JP, Hellmich B, et al. A vasculitis centre based management strategy leads to improved outcome in eosinophilic granulomatosis and polyangiitis (Churg–Strauss, EGPA): monocentric experiences in 150 patients. Annals of the Rheumatic Diseases. 2013; **72**(6):1011-1017. DOI: 10.1136/annrheumdis-2012-201531

Chapter 4

Capsule Endoscopy in Suspected and Established Small Bowel Crohn's Disease

Mauro Mastronardi and Elisabetta Cavalcanti

Abstract

Capsule endoscopy has recognized to be a very useful non-invasive tool for diagnosis and evaluation of the extension or the recurrence in Crohn's disease (CD) patients. It has the advantage of outstanding visualization of small-bowel lesions undetectable by conventional endoscopy or radiologic studies and has a good tolerability and safety in well-selected patients. In this chapter, we would like to evaluated the significant small bowel capsule endoscopy findings that can lead to better outcomes of diagnosis, classification, therapeutic management, and prognosis of patients with CD. Moreover, we would to discuss the specificity of the CE and to determine the place of the CE in the recurrence of CD and, for example, its role in monitoring drug response.

Keywords: capsule endoscopy, Crohn's disease, inflammatory bowel disease, small bowel investigation, medical devices

1. Introduction

Video capsule endoscopy (VCE) introduction and subsequent application in clinical practice almost 20 years ago [1], has revolutionized the management of a wide variety of small intestine diseases, allowing for the first time an extensive and high-quality examination of whole mucosal surface. VCE was minimally invasive, radiation-free and has an excellent safety profile. The most common indication for video capsule endoscopy is suspected a obscure gastrointestinal bleeding (OGIB), identification of small bowel malignant tumors, and follow-up of intestinal polyposis syndromes and the monitoring of mucosal inflammation in patients with active IBD in particular Crohn's disease (CD) as highlighted by several recent studies [2, 3]. VCE was able to detected even mildly inflammatory mucosal lesions, such as erythema, erosion, and small ulcers, which are rarely to highlight with radiological imaging modalities such as small bowel follow-through (SBFT), small bowel contrast ultrasound (SBCUS), CT enterography (CTE), and MR enterorrhaphy (MRE) [4, 5]. Yet, it lacks motion control and the possibility to perform biopsies or administer drugs. Hence the use of VCE has aided precision medicine-based diagnostic and therapeutic

 IntechOpen

decision-making, especially in patients with suspected or established Crohn's disease (CD) of the small intestine. Furthermore, in the last 20 years, its application has expanded allowing in patients with ulcerative colitis (UC), together with panenteric CD. This was made possible with the subsequent development of colonic capsule endoscopy (CCE), which allows visualization of both the small and large intestines [6, 7]. Therefore, the use of CE for the diagnosis and management of IBD is becoming more frequent and its implementation is considered a priority in the field of IBD. In this chapter, we would like to evaluated the significant small bowel capsule endoscopy findings that can lead to better outcomes of diagnosis, classification, therapeutic management, and prognosis of patients with CD. Moreover we would to discuss the specificity of the CE and to determine the place of the CE in the recurrence of CD and, for example, its role in monitoring drug response.

2. Video capsule endoscopy: type, technical and procedural aspects

Small bowel VCE was first introduced in 2000 as a noninvasive means of assessing the small bowel (SB) [1]. VCE, also known as wireless capsule endoscopy or video capsule endoscopy, is a gastrointestinal study that uses a pill camera to transmitted images of the intestinal lumen. The capsule was ingested orally, passed through passively via peristalsis and the images are downloaded from the data recorder to a computer for later review. The capsule was naturally eliminated from the body within 24 h, there was no need sedation or recovery time. At the present, several similar VCE systems are available worldwide, most of which wirelessly transmit and store images in an external recorder that patients carry during the recording. There are significant differences in the design of various CE systems (**Table 1**). Several small-bowel

	PillCam SB3 (Given Imaging Ltd., Israel).	**EndoCapsule System EC-1® (Olympus, Japan).**	**MiroCam® (IntroMedic, Korea).**	**OMOM (Chongqing Jinshan Science and Technology Group, China)**	**CapsoCam SV-1® (CapsoVision, Medical Innovations, US)**
Frame rate, fps	2–6	2	3	2	20 max
Dimension mm × mm	26.2 × 11.4	26 × 11	24.5 × 10.8	24.5 × 11	31 × 11
Battery life (h)	> 8	12	12	6–8	18–24 h
Transmission mode	RF	RF	RF	RF	USB
Field of view	156	145	160	140	360
Optical enanchament	FICE setting	Contrast setting	NA	NA	NA
FDA	Yes	Yes	Yes	No	No

Fps, frame per second; RF, radiofrequency; USB, universal serial bus; FICE, fujinon intelligent chromoendoscopy; NA, not applicable.
Given per Crohn (CE GINAm 2019).

Table 1.
Currently types of VCE available.

capsules (PillCam, Given Imaging, Yoqneam, Israel; EndoCapsule, Olympus, Tokyo, Japan; MiroCam, IntroMedic, Seoul, Korea; OMOM, Jinshan Science, Chongqing, China; CapsoCam, CapsoVision, Saratoga, CA, USA) are now available worldwide [8]. Capsule endoscope models with US FDA-approved capsule endoscope models include PillCam, EndoCapsule, and MiroCam. Although the various capsules are similar in size and shape, they differ in size, frame rate, runtime, field of view, image sensor, and optical enhancement. PillCam® is the original VCE and captures 2 frames per second. It has a "blood suspicious indicator" that can identify the site of bleeding. The third-generation capsule is about to be released, and almost all literature on VCE mentions PillCam. The EndoCapsule systems EC-1®, MiroCam® and OMOM are similar to the PillCam. The CapsoCam SV-1 is a new type of VCE with a 360 degree side view that does not require data loggers or sensors. Images are stored on the VCE itself, so the patient must remove the VCE from the stool. This VCE is then sent to the endoscope reader, which analyzes the data. It has a longer battery life of 18–24 h. Whether small bowel preparation is required for SBCE has been one of the most debated issues in capsule endoscopy science since the development of this diagnostic tool. The first manufacturer of small bowel capsule endoscopes recommended a low-fiber diet the day before surgery, drinking only water in the evening, followed by a 12-h fast, and advised against the use of laxatives before VCE. However, usually, 2 L polyethylene glycol (PEG) solution leads to improvement in small bowel visibility and diagnostic yield for SBCE [8]. Whether small bowel preparation is required for SBCE has been one of the most debated issues in capsule endoscopy science since the development of this diagnostic tool. The first manufacturer of small bowel capsule endoscopes recommended a low-fiber diet the day before surgery, drinking only water in the evening, followed by a 12-h fast, and advised against the use of laxatives before surgery. The choice of bowel preparation should be based on the patient's clinical situation. Patients should not take anything by mouth after midnight. On the morning of the capsule endoscopy, the patient should chew two simethicone tablets to reduce intraluminal air bubbles and improve visualization of the small bowel mucosa. The ideal dose of simethicone is yet to be defined and ranges between 80 and 200 mg [9]. After ingesting the video capsule, the patient needs to be nothing by mouth for at least 2 h. A clear liquid diet is allowed 2 h after capsule ingestion and light snack 4 h after capsule ingestion. Considering this evidence, the European Society of Gastrointestinal Endoscopy (ESGE) issued a technical review in 2018 recommending the use of purgative solutions prior to SBCE because the presence of residue in the small bowel lumen, limits observation, hampers interpretation, and may impair diagnostic accuracy [7]. Several meta-analyses confirmed that use of laxative solutions prior to SBCE improves small bowel cleansing but does not consensus has been reached regarding the optimal timing for purgative ingestion [10]. A meta-analysis of four randomized controlled trials (RCTs) highlighted that the use of prokinetics for capsule ingestion improves completion rate in SBCE [11]. Conversely, patients with incomplete SBCE studies were at increased risk (e.g., patients or subjects with one or more of the following: history of abdominal surgery, delayed gastric emptying, diabetic neuropathy, severe hypothyroidism, use psychotropic drugs, etc.) If the capsule remains in the stomach for more than 30–60 min, it may be affected by certain prokinetic drugs (metoclopramide or domperidone), as confirmed by real-time monitoring [12]. Probably the most relevant factor for attaining an adequate small bowel preparation is the timing and not the volume of the purgative solution. Many studies have now shown that factors other than the type of bowel preparation regime used, can influence the quality of bowel preparation among adult patients undergoing colonoscopy. These factors can be generally categorized as either patient-related (age, gender, co-morbidity, socioeconomic status) or procedure-related (adherence to bowel preparation instructions, timing of bowel preparation administration) [13]. Several authors reported that SBCE diagnostic yield is related with small bowel transit time (SBTT), with positive correlation between the diagnostic yield and SBTT, indicating that the longer the SBTT, the higher the diagnostic yield [14]. Proximal small bowel has a faster transit time and therefore, SBCE has a higher rate of missed lesions in this segment (ESGE 2018). Even though VCE guidelines was established, there were no formal recommendations and only limited data on how to increase performance and obtain a consistent level of high-quality reporting to guide capsule endoscopists on how to read the many images collected in each SBCE [15, 16]. In the following paragraphs we will be discussed the best to approach for VCE reading skills according to the management CD disease.

2.1 Patency capsule

The patency capsule (PC) is a dissolvable diagnostic tool, safe, efficient, and accurate for the assessment of the small intestine functional patency. PC reduces the risk of retention and allows the safe administration of a capsule endoscope. Even if it does not provide direct visual information for the presence and location of strictures, masses or narrowing of the lumen of the small intestine, its safe passage, in a pre-defined period of time minimizes the risk of retention and allows safe administration of a capsule endoscope.

The manufacturer company for the PillCamSB has developed a revolutionary system dubbed the Given® M2A Patency System. Its Patency capsule comprises of two timer plugs whose dissolving process initiates earlier (a mere 30 h after ingestion) and continues even when lodged in a tight stricture [17]. The patented Given and Agile patency capsules differ in composition (lactose for the Given capsule and dissolvable compounds with a radio frequency identification tag detectable by X-ray for Agile), number of timer plugs (1 for Given and 2 for Agile), and dissolution start time (40–100 h for Given and 30 h for Agile) [18].

Nowadays, there are two different approaches regarding PC administration in established CD: the selective approach (administering the PC only in patients with obstructing symptoms) and the nonselective approach (in all CD patients). The selective approach was warranted by the real-life retention risk of patients with established CD is 2.5%, a significantly lower probability compared with preliminary observations [19]. On the other hand, routine administration in patients with a low retention risk, such as patients under investigation for suspected CD without obstructive symptoms, known stenosis, or prior surgery, is not justified. Actually, the benefit of PC evaluation in selected patients with known or suspected CD was clear. Patency Capsule multi-center clinical trials [20, 21] highlighted the decreased risk of video capsule retention in patients with known strictures emphasizing that it was a valid and safe tool to assess functional patency of the small intestine. PC can identify those patients who can safely undergo capsule endoscopy, despite clinical and radiographic evidence of small bowel obstruction. The risk of PC-related adverse events was low. Abdominal pain, symptomatic PC retention/impaction, intestinal ischemia, cellophane wall impaction and aspiration were the most common complication that in most patients resolves spontaneously even if some go to medical, endoscopic, or surgical intervention for their management.

2.1.1 PC vs. other modalities

PC was as accurate in identifying stricture as or better than standard radiological techniques and was at least comparable to cross-sectional imaging methods. Although it cannot produce direct information on small bowel mucosal abnormalities; it should therefore be considered a complementary method to radiographic diagnostic methods—in particular, magnetic resonance (MR) imaging, specifically MR enteroclysis and MR enterography, reformed the investigation of CD small bowel involvement and related complications [22]. MR enterography was shown to be superior to MR enteroclysis, especially in the identification of minor lesions. an interesting study underlined that MR enteroclysis was an accurate method for the identification of small bowel strictures, [23] while MR enterography was shown to be highly sensitive (>90%) but moderately specific (52–59%) in the prediction of small bowel stenosis causing PC retention [24]. This is due to the interpretation of the results subject to the experience of the observer, preparation before the exam and among others the optimal ability of MR enterography to detect strictures areas is largely in the area of the terminal ileum. Although the PC only allows for assessment of the gut functional patency by not being able to discriminate between fibrostenotic and inflammatory strictures, although some studies suggest that it may allow the distinction between rigid and inflammatory strictures flexible fibrotic strictures [25]. Therefore, MR enterography could be really helpful in distinguishing between these two situations and predicting the feasibility of further investigations with PC and SBCE. However, However, PC offers a better assessment of functional intestinal patency than other noninvasive diagnostic modalities, particularly in the pediatric population [26]. In conclusion, PC was accurate in identifying stenosis as good as or better than standard radiological techniques but it cannot offer direct visual information regarding small bowel mucosa abnormalities and should be considered as a complementary method to radiographic diagnostic methods.

3. Diagnostic implication of capsule endoscopy in IBD

Crohn's disease (CD) and ulcerative colitis (UC) are chronic idiopathic and immune-mediated inflammatory bowel diseases (IBD) with a highly heterogeneous presentation and characterized by relapsing and remitting mucosal inflammation which mainly affects the gastrointestinal (GI) tract that necessitates lifelong monitoring and treatment. Most patients exhibit an inflammatory phenotype at diagnosis, but over time more than 50% of affected patients develop more serious chronic complications including strictures, fistulas, and/or abscesses, which in turn often require major surgery [27, 28]. Approximately 5–15% of patients cannot be classified as a subtype of IBD and the disease does not suitable the characteristic diagnostic criteria specific to either UC or CD. In these patients, the condition is labeled indeterminate colitis (IC) and inflammatory bowel disease unclassified (IBDU) [29]. The general assumption is that the diagnosis is provisional [30] until a more definitive diagnosis of UC or MC can be made. Therefore, patients with suspected or proven CD and IBDU must be evaluated frequently to assess or rule out SB lesions and the potential need for escalated care. In addition, it is reasonable to perform SB in patients with establishing RCU if clinical presentation changes or CD diagnoses was suspected. However, despite the advances, the diagnosis and management of IBD remain challenging. The establishment of new therapeutic goals, such as mucosal healing (MH) and the introduction of biologic therapies, based on tight monitoring and accelerated escalation of care, has created increasing demands and new indications for endoscopic assessment of disease activity [17–35]. These have been incorporated into the standard of care over the years, as are clinical guidelines developed by international societies such as the European Society for Gastrointestinal Endoscopy (ESGE) and the European Crohn's and Colitis Organization (ECCO) [28, 29]. In 2017, the American Gastroenterological Association (AGA) Institute Practice Guideline recommends SBCE for known, recurrent, or suspected Crohn's disease when active small bowel disease is suspected based on negative imaging studies and normal ileocolonoscopy.

Although these continue advance of novel indications, the SBCE was established to be principally a noninvasive instrument for the assessment of the SB mucosa that supports diagnosis and monitoring treatment of disease activity [36, 37], turning SBCE into a valuable decision-supporting tool.

3.1 Capsule endoscopy in suspected small bowel CD

Inflammatory disorders of the small bowel (SB) are frequently and can present in many different ways depending on the underlying cause such as Crohn disease, non-steroidal anti-inflammatory drug (NSAID) enteropathy, celiac disease, autoimmune enteropathy, radiation enteritis, infection and lymphoproliferative disorders.

CD was a chronic progressive inflammatory bowel disease that can affect any portion of the gastrointestinal tract, but affects the small intestine in up to 60% of cases [38].

Anyway, several SBCE findings are frequently associated with CD: aphthous lesions, serpiginous, linear or deep ulcerations, and mucosal edema (**Figure 1**). However, these findings are neither pathognomonic nonspecific to CD. Small-bowel

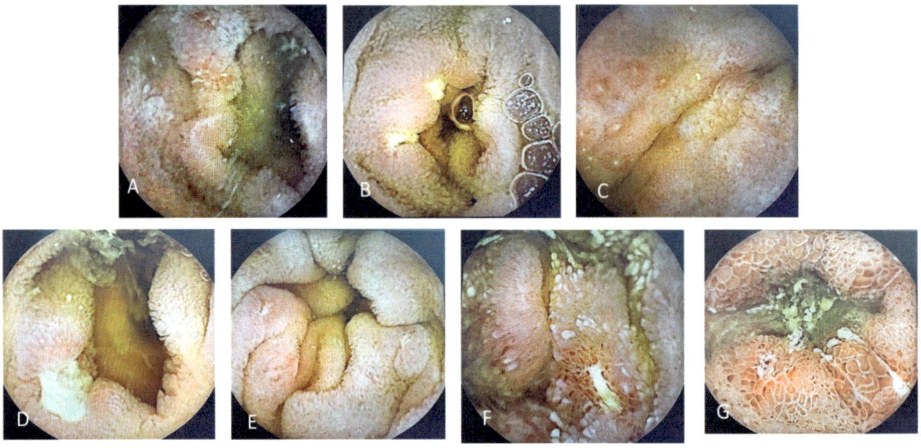

Figure 1.
Video capsule endoscopy for small bowel Crohn's disease. (A) Small and shallow aphtous ulcer in the duodenum were observered in suscpected CD patients, (B) small aphtous ulcer in the jejunum seen in suscpected CD patients, (C) apthous lesions in the distal jejunum were observed in suspected CD patients, (D) large ulcer in proximal ileal seen in established CD patients, (E) small erosion of the jejunum in established CD patients, (F) hiperemia, superficial ulceres and edematous mucosa in established CD patients and (G) edematous mucosa, hyperemia with extensive erosion and signs of bledding.

(SB) disease was involved in up to 80% of CD patients, while in about 30% of patients, the disease is limited to the SB exclusively [39, 40]. Small bowel CD was undervalued due to diagnostic limitations in visualizing the small bowel [41]. Small bowel CD is associated with serious complications such as strictures, abscesses, and obstruction. A gold standard for the diagnosis of CD is not available. CD has a multitude of phenotypes or presentations defined by the type, location, and disease severity. The diagnosis of Crohn's disease (CD) should be based on combined assessment of features of clinical history, symptoms, and evidence of intestinal inflammation based on imaging, endoscopy, histology, and biochemical parameters [42] Although ileocolonoscopy (IC) remains the primary modality for endoscopic evaluation in suspected cases [43].

3.1.1 Diagnostic yield and the clinical impact of SBCE

In Crohn's disease it is important to define the location of the disease.

Due to the length of the SB (average length of 575 cm at 20 years of age), the small bowel is difficult to examine directly and with conventional endoscopic equipment due to its complex loops and length [42]. Conventional endoscopic equipment can only be used to visualize the proximal jejunum and a small portion of the distal ileum. In particular SBCE could be appropriate to detect lesions outside the scope of conventional endoscopy because it seems to be more sensitive than imaging to detect a previously unrecognized disease location such as jejunal localization. Several studies have highlighted that jejunal disease was associated with an increased risk of structuring disease and abdominal surgeries as compared to either esophagogastroduodenal (EGD) or ileocolonic disease [44, 45]. Therefore, the CD distribution was crucial and upper gastrointestinal involvement was more frequent in children than in adults (30–80% vs 10–15%).

The Paris classification tried to avoid any ambiguity in the meaning of upper gastrointestinal lesions (L4) and further characterization of the L4 phenotype in the Montreal classification into three specific subgroups including L4-EGD, L4-jejunal, and L4-proximal ileal disease may be warranted [46]. A recent retrospective cohort study confirmed that L4 disease had a worse prognosis compared to non-L4 disease, and within L4 disease, the phenotype of L4-jejunal and L4-proximal ileal disease indicated a higher risk for intestinal surgery [47]. The most important comparative advantage of SBCE was considered its ability to visualize the small bowel and colonic mucosa directly and with higher sensitivity. Despite magnetic resonance enterography (MRE) has a good comparable diagnostic accuracy for small bowel disease, its presented a lower accuracy for mucosal inflammation. In the literature, SBCE has shown equal or higher diagnostic outcomes compared to MRE [48, 49]. Furthermore, SBCE was 50% diagnostic of CD when analyzed in a real setting [50]. Finally, the available magnetic resonance index of activity (MaRIA) has only been validated on the terminal ileum and colonic segments [51].

The role of SBCE for the detection of more proximal SB mucosal lesions is increasingly recognized. This is reflected in ECCO-ESGAR and ESGE guidelines and consensus statements [52]. A previous meta-analysis demonstrated that SBCE is a more sensitive method for the diagnosis of small bowel CD, with an incremental diagnostic yield 30% greater than other imaging modalities [48]. SBCE has a high sensitivity (93%) and a high negative predictive value (96%) for the diagnosis of small bowel CD [53, 54]. However, due to the high false positive rate and low specificity, SBCE should be used to exclude celiac disease rather than confirm it. Unfortunately, not all small bowel lesions are from CD, even after excluding the use of NSAIDs. A previous study showed that 14% of healthy individuals with SBCE [55]. Although various diagnostic modalities contribute to the diagnosis of CD, histopathological examination plays a key role. "Histopathology is not everything, but without histopathology we have nothing" [56, 57]. The presence of structural changes or "chronicity," such as crypt deformation, basal lymphoplasmacytosis, and metaplastic Paneth cells or pyloric glands, has been considered a prerequisite for the diagnosis of IBD, although these chronic structural changes are not characteristic of IBD. Conventional VCE or SBCE lack tissue sampling capabilities, so they are not suitable as sole diagnostic tests for CD or IBD. However, the limited invasiveness of SBCE may make it an inexpensive screening or adjunct test, providing a roadmap for targeted biopsy via routine enteroscopy, balloon-assisted enteroscopy, or IC. In this regard, disease biomarkers such as fecal calprotectin (FCP) could be useful in selecting patients for SBCE in suspected CD, as it helps exclude non-inflammatory small bowel lesions. Although measurement of these biomarkers offers a preliminary assessment of disease activity and can guide treatment decision-making regardless of disease location. However, their role in diagnosis MH (endoscopic remission) or predict treatment response was yet to be clarified. One study demonstrated that both FCP and C-reactive protein (CRP) had low negative predictive values for small bowel where Pan-intestinal video capsule endoscopy (PCE) observed mucosal inflammation among patients with normal biomarker levels [58].

A recent metanalysis underlined that a FCP cut off of more than 100 _g/g has highest diagnostic accuracy (sensitivity and specificity 73% and diagnostic odd ratio 7.89) [59]. Thus FCP was a selection tool for small bowel capsule endoscopy in suspected IBD with prior negative bi-directional endoscopy [60]. Therefore, careful mucosal assessment with SBCE has become pivotal to the diagnostic approach in patients with suspected CD. In summary, CD remains a difficult and challenging entity to manage. The suspected CD patient cohort presents a tough clinical scenario even after negative initial routine endoscopic investigations. SBCE has proven a high diagnostic yield and is often the preferred initial diagnostic test in suspected CD, because its noninvasive quality, better tolerance, and ability to view the entire small bowel. SBCE role was still uncertainty. This ambiguity is partly because of variations in the parameters used to diagnose CD using SBCE and the lack of a gold standard. Anyway, SBCE has a high negative predictive value in patients with suspected CD, making it an excellent "rule-out" test [61].

3.1.2 Role for repeat capsule endoscopy

A repeat capsule endoscopy may be useful for the evaluation of rebleeding, and/or unexplained gastrointestinal pain after a negative or nondiagnostic capsule endoscopy result. Due to the high diagnostic yield and noninvasive nature of CE, repeat CE remains a reasonable option due to patient acceptability and ease of use before other types of small bowel Studies have reported an incremental diagnostic yield of 35–75% with repeat capsule endoscopy and alteration in management in 39–62.5% of patients [55, 62]. When there is a high clinical suspicion for a small bowel tumor, CTE and/or deep enteroscopy may be preferred over a repeat capsule endoscopy. Viazis et al. [63] reported on 76 patients with new evidence of overt bleeding or a decrease in hemoglobin who underwent a second-look CE procedure. There were positive findings in 37 patients (49%) on second CE, findings of uncertain significance in 22 patients (29%) and 17 patients had no findings. The study concluded that certain patients would benefit from a second-look CE procedure. An interesting study [64] supported the hypothesis that repeat VCE is useful in equivocal and inconclusive studies where there is clinical suspicion of SB CD. The overall DY of CE recurrence in suspected SB-CD patients was 16.7% (3/18). However, patients without SB inflammation at the time of initial CE did not show any repeat CE indicates changes in CD (DY = 0). Patients with non-specific inflammation do not feel prompting CD in initial CE, DY in repeated CE was 33%. In addition, with higher fecal calprotectin results were more likely to provide evidences in support of a CD diagnosis in their repeat CE. In contrast, in patients whose initial CE showed no signs or evidence of SB inflammation, repeating the process does not seem to add much. Due to the high diagnostic yield and noninvasive nature of CE, repeat CE appears to be of benefit and should be considered for specific patients before other types of small bowel studies.

3.1.3 Role of pre-symptomatic and spondyloarthropathy patients

Spondyloarthritis (SpA) was a group of related chronic immune-mediated inflammatory disorders which share common genetic, pathophysiological and clinical features. IBD is a common extraintestinal manifestations in SpA patients, and around 8% of patients with ankylosing spondylitis develop clinically overt inflammatory bowel disease. Especially Crohn's disease percentage of 5–10% of patients with SpA that will develop inflammatory bowel disease and a much higher percentage, close to 60% of patients that have asymptomatic bowel inflammatory lesions [65]. Over 20 years ago, Mielants et al. [66] showed that a substantial number of these patients have subclinical ileal inflammation. Actually, approximately 50–60% of SpA patients display microscopic intestinal inflammation in biopsies of the ileum or colon, often reminiscent of Crohn's disease [67]. Since SpA and IBD patients share common genetic and immunopathogenic mechanisms [68], SpA patients have an up to four-fold increased risk of IBD compared to the general population. Different forms of SpA can be associated with variable frequencies of intestinal involvement, whereas articular involvement is frequently observed in IBD. Conventional endoscopic and radiological techniques are limited in their capacity to investigate the small bowel, thus often unable to detect CD mucosal lesions. CE uncovered SBI consistent with CD in 42.2% of patients with SpA, with a significant incremental yield over colonoscopy of 31% [69]. Significant small bowel findings (erythema, mucosal breaks, aphthous or linear ulcers, and erosions) were detected by capsule endoscopy in 30–80% of SpA patients [70]. Immunological link between SpA and IBD is still poorly understood. Even if there were relationship between the disease activity of SpA and the degree of gut inflammation [71]. A large percentage of SpA patients have subclinical gut inflammation without gastrointestinal symptoms and the presence of gut inflammation seems to be an important risk factor of progression of SpA [72]. Therefore in SpA patients when suspected IBD symptoms are present it's important to assessed the presence of small intestinal lesion using videocapsule endoscopy.

3.2 Capsule endoscopy in established CD

The management of IBD remains a challenge, indeed in the modern era of advanced biologic therapies. The need to differentiate between symptoms, endoscopic findings, and detecting of worsening disease activity at an early stage has set new goals in management. The approach to patients with suspected CD is different from the approach to patients with established CD. Although SBCE may have a limited role in the diagnosis of CD, it can be helpful in the assessment of a patient with known small bowel CD.

3.2.1 Diagnostic yield

SBVCE results impact clinical decision-making in a large cohort of patients with established CD. Previous studies have focused the definition of clinical impact in prognosis [73] and therapeutic changes [74, 75]. Although, the available scoring systems for quantification of SB inflammation (Lewis score and Capsule Endoscopy Crohn's Disease Activity Index) have not been extensively validated for the indication of monitoring of CD in large-scale clinical trials [76, 77]. Recent advances in the management of IBD have been a paradigm shift in treatment decisions for patients with established CD. In the past, the treatment was based mainly on the symptoms, but it is now known that symptoms were nonspecific for bowel inflammation. Actually, treatment strategies aim to treat beyond symptoms to normalization of objective markers of inflammation with the goal of mucosal healing. Mucosal healing at 1 year predicted an aggressive disease including the need for surgery.

Therefore, SBCE application in CD established can be regarded for assessment of disease activity, extent, severity, postoperative recurrence and mucosal healing once therapy was initiated.

Regarding mucosal healing, symptom assessment was a poor indicator of severity and extent of disease. In recent years, several studies have described the use of SBCE to monitor mucosal healing [78, 79] and postoperative recurrence [80].

Several studies have shown that SBCE can detect subtle mucosal abnormalities that other methods may miss.

SBCE can help identify CD missed by conventional endoscopy and assess the extent and severity of SB involvement [81]. Studies have also shown that the high diagnostic yield of SBCE affects disease management and clinical outcomes, thus hypothesizing that SBCE may play a role in assessing mucosal healing. In a prospective study of 28 patients with persistent symptoms, SBCE detected active inflammation in 82% of patients compared with ileocolonoscopy in only 49%, showing an incremental recovery of 33% [82].

Several recent studies evaluated the use of small bowel capsule endoscopy in the assessment of mucosal healing in patients diagnosed with Crohn's disease. Most of these studies did not evaluate a specific treatment, except for two studies, one of which focused on adalimumab and azathioprine [83] and the other that focused on certolizumab pegol [84]. In the other studies, there was no comparison between SBCE findings at baseline and during follow-up, because the most of patients in clinical remission had only one SBCE after treatment [85, 86]. Furthermore, according to these studies, the assessment of mucosal healing varies, although most of them are based on calculations of Lewis scores with normal values below 135. Overall, despite the high heterogeneity of these studies, the results suggest that mucosal healing can be assessed by SBCE to monitor the effect of drug therapy in CD patients, with a significant correlation between Lewis score and fecal calprotectin ($r = 0, 82$, $P < 0.0001$) [87], while there was no significant correlation between this score and clinical activity measured by CDAI [86].

Transmural healing (TH) is being increasingly recognized for reflecting deep remission in Crohn's disease. TH is an independent predictor of more favorable long-term outcomes than MH, suggesting that TH could become the potential treatment endpoint in CD [88]. In the future it will be important to evaluate transmural healing rather than MH, currently SBCE only detects MH so in the future to define disease remission SBCE will have to be integrated with the use of transversal imaging for established CD.

ECCO topical review (2018) recommends an appropriate reevaluation of disease activity considering clinical, biochemical, endoscopic and/or radiological techniques before withdrawing treatment of SBCE may play a key role in this regard. Mucosal healing in SBCE was the only independent factor predicting treatment downgrade in logistic regression. A remission as measured by the Harvey-Bradshaw index or inflammatory markers within this range, such as FCP or CRP, was not associated with discontinuation of treatment. Indeed, to assess remission endoscopic evaluation it was needs an endoscopic assessment for a appropriate risk evaluation and cannot rely on indirect parameters.

In patients with quiescent Crohn's disease involving the small bowel, fecal calprotectin predicts short term flare risk, whereas VCE predicts both short-term and long-term risk of disease exacerbation. In particular Shomron Ben-Horin et al. [89] underlined that VCE can identify patients who are at high risk of flare within 24 months, whereas fecal calprotectin can only identify patients who are at high risk of flare within 3 months. If supported by additional studies, protocols incorporating VCE could expand the scope of available methods for monitoring disease activity and predicting outcomes in small bowel Crohn's disease.

However, the definition of endoscopic remission as assessed by SBCE remains unknown because there is currently no consensus on the therapeutic objective to reach in luminal SB CD (normalization of SBCE or absence of deep or superficial ulcerations).

3.2.2 Comparison with other modalities

After CD is diagnosed, the extent of disease throughout the gastrointestinal tract should be determined.

Current practice uses MRE, which allows transmural visualization of the small bowel without exposing the patient to ionizing radiation and its potential future complications, or involving invasive procedures. However, SBCE can identify small bowel lesions that may not be detected by MRI. Although most guidelines do not recommend SBCE in patients with normal MRE or CTE [90], it can be considered for certain indications such as anemia, malnutrition and discrepancy between symptoms and instrumental investigations In patients with established CD, a meta-analysis of various modalities used in small bowel CD showed SBCE was superior to barium studies (small bowel follow-up or enema) (38%; 95% CI, 22–54%; $P < 0.00001$) and CTE (32%; 95% CI, 16–47%; $P < 0.0001$)) but not ileoscopy (13%; 95% CI, −1 to 26%; P 1/4 0.07) or MRE (−6%; 95% CI, −30% to 19%; P 1/4 0.65) [91]. It has been suggested that MRE may be superior to CTE in detecting strictures and strengthening of the ileal wall MRE and CTE have been shown to play an important role in established CD. Wall thickening and abnormal enhancement were sensitive indicators of CD, whereas abnormal T2 signal, mesenteric vascular prominence, and adenopathy were specific. It has been suggested that MRE may be superior to CTE in detecting strictures and strengthening of the ileal wall. Regarding MRE, a valid index based on wall thickness, relative contrast enhancement, edema, and ulceration has been developed, called Magnetic Resonance Activity Index (MaRIA) [92]. Recent advances in the management of IBD have been a paradigm shift in treatment decisions for patients with established CD. In the past, the treatment was based mainly on the symptoms, but it is now known that symptoms were nonspecific for bowel inflammation. There was still controversy about the most optimal way to evaluate SB inflammation.

In a prospective study [93] of patients with CD experiencing mild/no clinical symptoms, VCE was better tolerated compared to MRE and was preferred by 78% of patients due to less side effects. [94] VCE is also able to detect more cases of proximal SB CD than MRE.

In this case SBCE was helpful for prognostic purposes because proximal CD is associated with higher risk of stricture formation and need for surgical intervention.

Early identification of this high-risk group may allow for earlier aggressive therapy to reduce risk of CD complications. Besides, SBCE played a key role in persistent clinical suspicion despite negative ileocolonscopy and cross-sectional imaging. In a prospective study of patients with persistent perianal disease but negative standard work-up, VCE had an incremental diagnostic yield of 24% following negative ileocolonoscopy and radiology imaging [95].

Although the accuracy of SBCE in monitoring proximal SB-CD has not been formally compared with device-guided enteroscopy due to the invasive nature of the latter procedure, the mucosal changes in distal SB observed with CE appear to be comparable to those observed with ileocolonoscopy standard modality for evaluating changes in terminal ileum CD [96]. The diagnostic superiority of SBCE over radiography has also been demonstrated in patients with established CD. In earlier meta-analyses, CE vs. SB barium studies (71% vs. 36%; IY 5 38%; 95% CI, 22–54%) and CT enterography/bowel lavage (71% vs. 39%, IJ 5 32%, 95% CI, 16–47%), Although the accuracy of SBCE in monitoring proximal SB-CD has not been formally compared with device-guided enteroscopy due to the invasive nature of the latter procedure, the mucosal changes in distal SB observed with CE appear to be comparable to those observed with ileocolonoscopy. Consistent, reference standard, associated with terminal ileum CD [97]. The diagnostic superiority of SBCE over radiography has also been demonstrated in patients with established CD. In earlier meta-analyses, CE vs. SB barium studies (71% vs. 36%; IY 5 38%; 95% CI, 22–54%) and CT enterography/bowel lavage (71% vs. 39%, IJ 5 32%, 95% CI, 16–47%), but not when related with MR enteroclysis/enterography (70% vs. 79%; IY 5 6%; 95% CI, 30–19%) [98]. In a recent analysis of studies comparing SBCE diagnostic rates with radiological techniques, Kopylov and colleagues [99] underlined a modest correlation between SBCE and MRE-based quantitative indices of inflammation in patients with quiescent SB CD. Between-modality correlation was higher in patients with endoscopically severe disease.

Despite several modality-specific limitations, both SBCE and MRE provide an accurate and comprehensive assessment of SB and are capable of detecting persistent inflammation in most patients with clinically quiescent disease. The agreement between patterns was significantly better in patients with overt SB inflammation.

Therefore, SBCE and cross-sectional imaging (MRE and CT) are complementary diagnostic tools in CD established. In established non stricturing CD patients, SBCE was able to detect fine mucosal lesions especially in the proximal SB. Instead, cross-sectional imaging can detect more severe disease activity and better characterize the CD phenotype in terms of extraluminal involvement. Another retrospective study highlighted a significantly higher sensitivity of SBCE in detecting proximal and distal disease in the small bowel (jejunum and ileum) compared to MRE (76.6% vs. 44.7% $p = 0.001$) [5]. Compared with partial small bowel visualization endoscopy that occurs during endoscopy, SBCE exhibits high sensitivity to minor erosions or defects in the intestinal mucosa changes below the detection threshold of the imaging modality, and high sensitivity to small bowel length coverage.

However, if only one MRE or CE test can be performed during follow-up, there are limitations to the results each technique can provide. Therefore, it is necessary to recognize the advantages and disadvantages of these test methods. In particular, **Table 2** summarized and compared three diagnostic modalities.

3.2.3 Retention and management of retained capsule

VCE is a relatively safe and well-tolerated procedure. There are, however, a few limitations. However, certain complications arise as a result of the procedure, and they have been divided into clinical and technical complications (**Table 3**). The most important and common clinical complications was capsule retention in the gut lumen. Capsule retention can affect any area of the digestive system and remains undetected for a minimum of 2 weeks unless removed surgically or endoscopically. Most of the patients remain asymptomatic and in about one-third, the capsule is naturally excreted later than 15 days after ingestion [100, 101].

In a large multicenter retrospective study of CE-related adverse events, 61.5% of patients remained asymptomatic despite retention, 37.5% of events resolved spontaneously after a median of 42 days, and 19.2% of events passed after a median of 24 days medication resolved [93]. Nevertheless, in some patients acute obstruction or intestinal perforation has been reported [102–104]. This is a major worry not just for patients but also for physician. The overall incidence of capsule retention is low, approximately 1–2%. Thankfully, meta-analysis covering 227 publications and 22,840

	Capsule endoscopy	MR enterography	CT enterography
Advantage	Endoscopic view may detect subtle lesion Superior proximal SB lesion detection	Extraluminal finding	Extraluminal finding Widespread availability
Disadvantage	Risk of capsule retention and bowel obstruction Distal small bowel view may be obscured by debris	Long scan time in tight space (claustrophobia) Intravenous contrast Metal foreign object contraindicated Underdistention of bowel loops can compromise view	Ionizing radiation Intravenous contrast

Table 2.
Advantages and disadvantages of capsule endoscopy versus MR enterography versus CT enterography.

Clinical complications	Capsule retention Failure to reach the ileocecal valve—incomplete examination of the small bowel Swallowing disorders—inability to swallow and/or aspiration of the device.
Technical complications	Gaps in the recordings Short duration of capsule batteries Malfunction of battery pack Failure to activate the capsule Failure of localization software Failure of downloading Bowel preparation

Table 3.
Complications of capsule endoscopy.

capsule studies reported an overall retention rate of 1.4%, compared with the overall incidence retention rate of 2.6% for established CD [105]. This higher rate of retention can be attributed to the increased likelihood of intestinal strictures in CD. Risk of capsule retention can be stratified using cross-sectional imaging such as MRE/CTE or patency capsule, both of which have high negative predictive value, and can lower the overall risk of retention to 2.7% (95% CI, 1.1–6.4%) [21]. Nonselective use of patency capsule in all patients with established CD did not reduce the rate of capsule retention compared with a selective approach based on history of obstructive symptoms, previous obstruction, or previous abdominal surgery [106]. Symptomatic intestinal obstruction due to patency capsule is rare and usually managed conservatively [107]. The disadvantage of patency capsule testing is false positive rate which can be reduced by low dose, spot computed tomography, which can determine the exact location of capsule. False positive results are often due to colonic retention as a result of prolonged transit times. This can significantly reduce false positive patency tests. ESGE recommends that in asymptomatic patients without intestinal obstruction, capsule retention be initially treated conservatively with drugs (e.g., laxatives, prokinetics, steroids, immunomodulators, and biologics). If that fails, enteroscopy with a capsule retrieval device should be performed. If enteroscopy fails to recover the capsule; the next step is surgery (laparoscopy or open surgery with enterotomy) to remove the capsule (ESGE 2015). Another clinicals complication was the incomplete examination of the small bowel means that the capsule has not reached the cecum. Rodonotti et al. [108] in a retrospective analysis of 733 consecutive examinations underlined that failure to reach the ileocecal valve occurred approximatively in 15% of cases. In most cases the causes may be the failure to enter the duodenum with the capsule remaining in the stomach for the entire recording time, the delay in passing the pylorus and the retention of the capsule. These complications prevented or hindered the diagnosis in 38%. An increased risk of gastric retention and delayed gastric transit time should be suspected in patients who have diabetes, prior vagotomy, or scleroderma [109]. A prokinetic agent may be administered before the start of the examination to reduce the risk of this complication.

Swallowing disorders are a relative contraindication to capsule endoscopy. Possible complications related to swallowing the capsule include inability to swallow and/or aspiration of the device. Accidental Capsule endoscope aspiration into the respiratory tract is a rare complication of capsule endoscopy. The incidence of capsule aspiration in a large cohort of patients was very low. Rare case reports reported it may cause life threatening acute respiration distress, and over half of patients required bronchoscopy intervention after capsule aspiration [110, 111]. A meta-analysis study reported that aspiration was observed only in 2 out of 5.428 patients resulting in an incidence of 0.003% [112]. However, in some cases, induced shortness of breath necessitates removal of the aspirated capsule via bronchoscopy using general anesthesia. There is no established method to accurately predict and thus prevent capsule endoscope aspiration. Lack of symptoms associated with capsule inhalation can be dangerous as the capsule may remain in the airway until visualized on video, resulting in potentially life-threatening adverse event including respiratory failure [113]. Therefore, in elderly patients and in cases where capsule swallowing is difficult or symptomatic, post-capsule observation in real-time as possible is strongly recommended. Capsule aspiration should be considered an emergency. The presence of dysphagia is a relative contraindication to capsule endoscopy.

Most common technical complications were as short-life capsule batteries, downloading failure, failure of the localization software, recording gaps and inability to activate the capsule. A review of 733 VCE studies underlined those technical limitations and failures were encountered in a small number of cases, mainly in the initial phase of capsule use and have been largely overcome with the use of improved equipment.

A more serious problem was the inability to download endoscopic images from the recorder to the workstation, hampering inspection and diagnosis of the records. Again, this problem occurred in only 5 cases (0.68%), limited to the early experience of each center. Overall, technical limitations prevented the diagnosis in 21/63 examinations (Rondotti 2005). Although the technology of capsule endoscopy has made significant progress, there are rare technical limitations and failures that hindered or prevented the diagnosis in a small number of cases.

One of the disadvantages of capsule endoscopy was the inability to maneuver the device and difficult to adjust the field of view as desired, stopping at a certain area for diagnostic or therapeutic purposes. It was also difficult to return to an area, re-observe, to accurately measure the lesion's size and to do biopsies. The overall miss rates of SBCE for small bowel tumors and ulcers were 18.9% and 0.5%, respectively [114]. These shortcomings can be overcome by adding the Magnetic assisted capsule endoscopy (MACE). MACE exanimated the gastrointestinal tract by control the location of the capsule endoscope swallowed by the patient using a magnetic field in real-time. The magnetic field generated outside the human body makes it possible to adjust a capsule endoscope equipped with a permanent magnet [115].

Finally, another limitation of using SBCE is the time it takes to read the results. Reliable and rapid reading of SBCE images remains a challenge, leading to missed lesions and inter-personal variability in interpreting results. Various software applications have been developed in recent years with the aim of reducing reading time by automatically selecting and interpreting images for diagnostic CDs (Quick view, top 100 images, Atlas). In addition, the use of artificial intelligence (AI) in medicine was rapidly progressing. In a recent review of AI applications in gastroenterology, various models have been analyzed in inflammatory lesions or gastrointestinal bleeding during wireless SBCE, demonstrating a high level of precision for disease detection [116]. This might represent a remarkable step forward in reducing the reading time. The efficacy of such technologies in IBD remains to be proven [51]. Therefore, the consideration reported in this carapter should be careful for further discussion and validation Despite these limitations, the NGT process is a valid method to systematically identify and prioritize ideas behind PCE for monitoring established CD. The role of SBCE for monitoring established CD in terms of target patient populations and benefits compared to other diagnostic modalities was undisputed. SBCE was an efficient method in a "treat-to-target" strategy for CD management and to prioritize efforts in further research needs. Future studies should focus on comparing the SBCE-guided approach to standard of care for all patients with established CD and involvement of both the colon and small bowel and should consider clinical, patient-reported, and economic outcomes.

4. Role in postoperative CD

In evaluating recurrence in patients with CD who underwent surgery, SBCE showed superior yield than ileocolonoscopy (62% vs. 25%), with the advantage of detecting proximal small bowel lesions. It is difficult to pass a surgical anastomosis and observe the proximal part by ileocolonoscopy in patients who underwent side-to-side reconstitution of a neoiluem, which is why CE is more useful [117].

SBCE is also make use to diagnose recurrences of CD after surgery and VCE might increase diagnostic accuracy and impact therapeutic decisions.

After ileocolonic resection, clinical or surgical recurrence was frequently preceded by endoscopic recurrence of the neo terminal ileum in up to 70% of patients. Ileal lesions can be scored by Rutgreet's score at the first ileocolonoscopy (ideally at 6 months postoperatively) The Rutgeerts score (RS) was established to predict post operative recurrence and to lead medical therapy. However, this scoring system groups ileal and anastomotic injuries into the same category. A modified RS was developed to separate isolated anastomotic lesions and those in the neo-terminal ileum to further understand the role of anastomotic lesions in CD progression [80, 118]. Although ileo-colonoscopy was the standard method to diagnose postoperative CD recurrence, recent findings suggest that VCE was less sensitive in detecting recurrence in the neo-terminal ileum. However, VCE can identify two-thirds of the lesions that ileo-colonoscopy cannot reach [80]. Furthermore, studies indicated that ileal recurrence, rather than anastomotic recurrence, was a better predictor of CD's long-term outcomes [119]. As such in postoperative CD, VCE has the potential to improve clinical outcomes beyond the scope of ileo-colonoscopy.

5. Role in IBD unclassified

VCE plays a significant role in inflammatory bowel disease type unclassified (IBDU) since it provides visualization throughout the small bowel and contributes to its reclassification. A Lewis score of over 95% has a 90% sensitivity and 100% specificity in diagnosing CD [120].

In patients with IBDU, VCE can identify newly emerged small bowel lesions, which correspond to CD, in approximately 29–40% of cases [121]. This was particularly significant in pediatric IBD and can greatly influence treatment decisions [122]. Although VCE has high sensitivity to rule out small bowel involvement, up to 20% IBD-U patients with normal VCE can develop new small bowel lesions suggestive of CD on follow up.

Moreover, it is important to make a prompt diagnosis of IBD, it is equally important not to misdiagnose IBD. Since, there are many differential diagnoses which may have a similar presentation to IBD endoscopically, thus any significant findings on SBCE should be followed up with enteroscopy and biopsies according to ESGE Guideline (2023).

Furthermore, small bowel ruptures into the mucous membranes/lesions are common and asymptomatic and can lead to overdiagnosis of IBD. Besides, it is important to evaluate the role of SBCE on the reclassification of colonic inflammatory bowel disease type unclassified (IBDU). An interesting retrospective study [123] including patients with IBDU undergoing SBCE was objectively assessed by determining the Lewis score (LS). SBCE lead to reclassification of disease from IBDU to definitive CD in 25% of cases. Although a negative SBCE study did not allow to definitely exclude a future diagnosis of small bowel CD, as further investigation and biopsies on follow-up led to a diagnosis of CD in one patient, the absence of significant inflammatory activity (LS < 135) in the small intestine actually allowed exclusion of CD in 94% of cases.

The correct diagnosis of inflammatory bowel disease is extremely important to define prognosis, therapeutic orientation and surgical intervention.

6. Scoring systems

Nevertheless, there is a current lack of integrated evidence to guide optimal monitoring in terms of appropriate tools and timing Surveillance of established Crohn's disease through a "treat-to-target" strategy aimed at reducing and preventing long-term bowel damage and disability. Despite the availability of various monitoring techniques, comprehensive evidence for optimal monitoring in terms of appropriate tools and timing is currently lacking. In particular, whole-bowel video capsule endoscopy (PCE) allows noninvasive and direct visualization of the entire bowel, and its safety and efficacy have been demonstrated [51].

In this setting, SBCE may be particularly helpful in supporting decisions about escalating treatment for CD with persistent symptoms. In this case, a negative SBCE study indicates that symptoms are likely due to other non-inflammatory causes, such as IBD or bacterial overgrowth. If the test is positive, it is important to consider that the poor specificity and interobserver agreement of SBCE may lead to overtreatment of celiac disease in this setting. The Capsule Endoscopy Small Bowel CD Activity Index assessed inflammation, anatomic extent, and the presence of strictures was prospectively validated in a multicenter study. Finally, SBCE has also shown promise in postoperative recurrence monitoring, with excellent sensitivity but relatively low specificity compared with other modalities, including colon ultrasound and MRE [124]. Given the risks of capsule retention and the inability to obtain tissue samples, CE is unlikely to replace ileocolonoscopy as standard practice in patients undergoing ileocolectomy. However, it may still play a role in patients undergoing SB resection and entero-intestinal anastomosis inaccessible by standard endoscopy. An objective clinical activity score is recommended to assess disease severity, small bowel involvement, and response to drug therapy.

To determine disease severity, small bowel involvement and response to medical treatment, it's recommended to utilize objective clinical activity scores. It's important to note that while these scores can assess the type, location and severity of small bowel involvement, they cannot be utilized for diagnosing small bowel CD. The recent ESGE and ECCO guidelines supported the use of endoscopic activity scores for the classification of inflammatory activity in patients with CD undergoing SBCE, such as the Lewis score or the Capsule Endoscopy Crohn's Disease Activity Index (CECDAI) [52]. CECDAI, which evaluates inflammation severity, disease extent and stenosis, is a simpler alternative to LS and has been shown to be more reflective of active small bowel inflammation in comparative studies [125]. Although there's a strong correlation between LS and CECDAI, only moderate correlation was observed with stool biomarkers such as fecal calprotectin. A recent study found a LS range of 135–790 to be equivalent to a CECDAI score of 4.9–6.9.

The recent ESGE and ECCO guidelines supported the use of endoscopic activity scores for the classification of inflammatory activity in patients with CD undergoing SBCE, such as the Lewis score or the CECDAI. It is unclear whether these indexes are interchangeable for the evaluation of mucosal inflammation in established Crohn's disease.

The Lewis score (LS) was developed to differentiate between significant and nonsignificant inflammation of the intestine, as well as to assess inflammatory activity [126]. In particular, LS is based upon distribution and presence of ulcers villous edema and stenosis. The LS divided the small bowel into three equal tertiles (by small bowel transit time) and for each tertile, villous edema and ulcers are assessed based on its characteristics and extension. The final score results of the sum of the tertiles with the highest score for villous edema and ulcers, plus the stenoses score rated for the whole examination It consists of dividing the SB into 3 equal parts (tertiles) based on SB capsule transit time and assigning a sub- score to each tertile based on the degree of edema or ulceration. The sum of the worst affected tertile is then added to a stenosis score (**Table 4**). LS score in the reading software for the automatic calculation has been incorporated into PillCam platfor. A score < 135 indicates normal or clinically insignificant mucosal inflammatory changes, 135–790 indicates mild inflammation, and a score ≥ 790 indicates moderate-to-severe inflammation. The application of LS ≥135 as the cutoff value for the presence of significant inflammatory activity in patients undergoing SBCE for suspected CD may be useful to establish the diagnosis of CD. Based on assessments of villous edema, ulcers, and stenosis, the LS classifies CD activity from mild to severe. The SBCE detects nonspecific lesions of CD, and the LS assesses the grade of inflammatory activity regardless of the etiology. In literature a series of study [127, 128] including patients with suspected CD submitted to SBCE and with a large period of follow-up after the capsule underlined that the application of LS ≥135 as the cutoff value for the presence of significant inflammatory activity in patients undergoing SBCE for suspected CD has a high sensitivity and specificity and may be useful to establish the diagnosis, when integrated with other relevant diagnostic elements.

The CECDAI or Niv score is another prospectively validated scoring system.

CECDAI assesses the severity of inflammation, stenosis, and the extent of disease (**Table 5**). In a comparison study, CECDAI emerged as a simpler and more accurate indicator of active small bowel inflammation than LS [55]. CECDAI was validated in multicenter prospective study of patients with isolated small-bowel CD [129], summing up the score in the proximal and distal portions of SB (based on transit time) across the three endoscopic parameters:: inflammation (A, 0 to 5 points), extent of disease (B, 0 to 3 points), and strictures (C, 0 to 3 points), both for the proximal and distal 10 segments of the small bowel based on the transit time of the capsule (**Table 3**). Even if no clear cut-off for inflammatory severity has been validated for the CECDAI score, the values of 3.8 and 5.8 correlate approximately to the 135 and

Parameters	Number	Longitudinal extent	Descriptors
Villous appearance	Normal—0	Short segment—8	Single—1
	Edematous—1	Long segment—12	Patchy—14
	>8	Whole tertile—20	Diffuse—17
Ulcer	None—0	Short segment—5	<1/4– 9
	Single—3	Long segment—10	1/4–1/2–12
	Few—5	Whole tertile—15	>1/2–18
	Multiple—10		
Stenosis (rated for the whole study)			
Stenosis	None—0	Ulcerated—24	Traversed—7
	Single—14	Non-ulcerated—2	Not traversed—10
	Multiple—20		
Lewis score = tertile with highest score (result of oedema and ulcers) plus score of stenosis for the entire small bowel.			

Table 4.
Lewis score.

Parameters	Score
A. Inflammation score	0 = None
	1 = Oedema/hyperaemia/denudation (mild to moderate)
	2 = Oedema/hyperaemia/denudation (severe)
	3 = Bleeding, exudate, aphthae, erosion, ulcer <0.5 cm
	4 = Ulcer 0.5–2 cm, pseudopolyp
	5 = Large ulcer >2 cm
B. Extent of disease score	0 = No disease (normal examination)
	1 = Focal disease (single segment
	2 = Patchy disease (2–3 segments)
	3 = Diffuse disease (>3 segments)
C. Stricture score	None – 0
	1 = Single-passed
	2 = Multiple-passed
	3 = Obstruction (non-passage)
Segmental score (proximal or distal) = (A × B) + C	
Total score = **proximal** [(A × B) + C + **distal** (A × B) + C]	

Table 5.
CECDAI (Niv score) for capsule endoscopy.

790 cut-offs of the Lewis score, respectively. Lastly, measuring the extent and severity of inflammation is important in established small bowel CD as a "Treat to target" strategy based on mucosal healing can reduce disease related complications leading to surgery and hospitalization. SBCE could be useful for refining disease location and prognosis, assessing mucosal healing in patients receiving treatment, and monitoring patients in the post-operative setting.

7. Capsule endoscopy and artificial intelligence

An important limitation to the applicability of VCE in daily practice is the substantial time required to review images acquired during capsule endoscopy. Artificial intelligence (AI) is being tested to reduce review time and obtain accurate diagnoses without missing any lesions. Deep learning-based methods, especially convolutional neural networks (CNN), have been used in capsule endoscopy to detect bleeding, vasodilation, ulcers, cancer, and hookworms. The sensitivity and accuracy in detecting these lesions is close to 100% [125]. The AI model proved effective in detecting colorectal polyps or tumors, achieving high sensitivity of 47.4–98.1% and high specificity of 87.0%–96.3% in each frame analysis [130]. An evolution of AI research is capsule endoscopy (CE), with several publications evaluating the role of deep learning in automatic detection of inflammatory lesions, vascular lesions, [131–133] herniated and neoplastic lesions/mass, and assessment of bowel cleanliness [134]. However, many challenges remain to translate the impressive experimental capabilities of AI in CE into clinical practice. Some of these challenges include standardizing results, validating established endpoints, creating common datasets and computational methods, and linking to clinical outcomes. These challenges are in part common to other areas of gastrointestinal endoscopy and general medicine [135]. In recent studies [136] all methods and study designs used were heterogeneous. Therefore, a formal meta-analysis of all literature studies could not be performed. Most studies have limited sample sizes and cannot test the performance of their AI models. Especially for research using machine learning or deep learning, a large fraction of CCE images is required to train the model, which limits the number of remaining images to test the model. Practical implementation of AI review of CCE-2 colon images was a critical step towards the applicability of CCE in daily clinical practice. In order to be able to fully assess the added value of the AI method, the study should always indicate the version of the capsule used and the accuracy of its model in terms of sensitivity and specificity. Furthermore, studies would be better off using only results from experienced CCE readers to test the performance of their AI methods, as the sensitivity and specificity of findings represent the ability of AI models to achieve the same level of performance as these readers. There is no doubt that AI has potential benefits for both physicians and patients, but applying it to clinical practice is challenging. While the U.S. Food and Drug Administration (FDA) has approved some assistive algorithms, there are currently no guidelines specific to AI's role in disability [137].

8. Conclusion

SBCE was safe, highly sensitive but not specific for detection of mucosal inflammation in small bowel CD [138]. SBCE played a pivotal role in suspected and established CD (**Figure 2**) and its was a useful tool for approaching therapeutic management in CD patients both for treatment escalation and de-escalation.

Therefore, in suspected CD with negative ileo-colonoscopy, SBCE was a reliable diagnostic tool for assessment in the absence stenotic lesions that prevent its passage and thus necessitate further invasive diagnostic modalities. Hence, fecal calprotectin

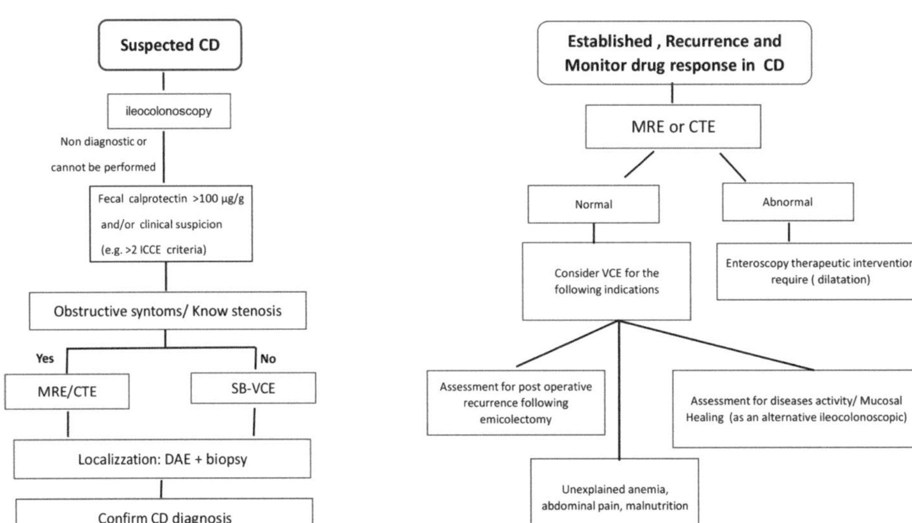

Figure 2.
Suggested diagnostic algorithm for the use of small bowel capsule endoscopy in CD.

can be used as a tool for selecting patients with suspected small bowel CD for SBCE. In the presence of obstructive symptoms or known stenosis, MRE/CTE should be preferred over VCE given the high risk of capsule retention.

In established CD, SBCE can help in detecting precise disease location, disease severity, monitoring response to therapy and mucosal healing. In post-operative SB disease, SBCE may be helpful to evaluate recurrence. After 20 years since its introduction, with all the above knowledge in mind, it is plausible to conclude that utilization of SBCE is safe if current indications are respected and it has significantly contributed to the knowledge of pathologies of the small bowel and to their therapy, through the production of a florid and large amount of scientific literature.

Author details

Mauro Mastronardi and Elisabetta Cavalcanti*
Department of Gastroenterology of National Institute of Gastroenterology IRCCS "S. de Bellis", Bari, Italy

*Address all correspondence to: elisabetta.cavalcanti@irccsdebellis.it

References

[1] Iddan G, Meron G, Glukhovsky A, Swain P. Wireless capsule endoscopy. Nature. 2000;**405**:417. DOI: 10.1038/35013140

[2] Rondonotti E, de Franchis R. Diagnosing coeliac disease: Is the videocapsule a suitable tool? Digestive and Liver Disease. 2007;**39**:145-147. DOI: 10.1016/j.dld.2006.10.005

[3] Pennazio M, Rondonotti E, de Franchis R. Capsule endoscopy in neoplastic diseases. World Journal of Gastroenterology. 2008;**14**:5245-5253. DOI: 10.3748/wjg.14.5245

[4] Hong SM, Jung SH, Baek DH. Diagnostic yields and clinical impacts of capsule endoscopy. Diagnostics. 2021;**11**:1842. DOI: 10.3390/diagnostics11101842

[5] González-Suárez B, Rodriguez S, Ricart E, Ordás I, Rimola J, Díaz-González Á, et al. Comparison of capsule endoscopy and magnetic resonance enterography for the assessment of small bowel lesions in Crohn's disease. Inflammatory Bowel Diseases. 2018;**24**:775-780. DOI: 10.1093/ibd/izx107

[6] Eliakim R, Fireman Z, Gralnek IM, Yassin K, Waterman M, Kopelman Y, et al. Evaluation of the PillCam Colon capsule in the detection of colonic pathology: Results of the first multicenter, prospective, comparative study. Endoscopy. 2006;**38**:963-970. DOI: 10.1055/s

[7] Rondonotti E, Spada C, Adler S, May A, Despott EJ, Koulaouzidis A, et al. Small-bowel capsule endoscopy and device-assisted enteroscopy for diagnosis and treatment of small-bowel disorders. European Society of Gastrointestinal Endoscopy (ESGE) Technical Review Endoscopy. 2018;**50**(4):423-446. DOI: 10.1055/a-0576-0566

[8] Koulaouzidis A, Rondonotti E, Karargyris A. Small-bowel capsule endoscopy: A ten-point contemporary review. World Journal of Gastroenterology. 2013;**19**:3726-3746. DOI: 10.3748/wjg.v19.i24.3726

[9] Albert J, Gobel CM, Lesske J, Lotterer E, Nietsch H, Fleig WE. Simethicone for small bowel preparation for capsule endoscopy: A systematic, single-blinded, controlled study. Gastrointestinal Endoscopy. 2004;**59**(4):487-491. DOI: 10.1016/S0016-5107(04)00003-3

[10] Xavier S, Rosa B, Monteiro S, Arieira C, Magalhães R, Gonçalves TC, et al. Bowel preparation for small bowel capsule endoscopy—The later, the better! Digestive and Liver Disease. 2019;**51**(10):1388-1391

[11] Koulaouzidis A, Giannakou A, Yung DE, Dabos KJ, Plevris JN. Do prokinetics influence the completion rate in small-bowel capsule endoscopy? A systematic review and meta-analysis. Current Medical Research and Opinion. 2013;**29**(9):1171-1185. DOI: 10.1185/03007995.2013.818532

[12] Emanuele R et al. Small-bowel capsule endoscopy and device-assisted enteroscopy: ESGE technical review. Endoscopy. 2018;**50**:423-446

[13] Romero RV, Mahadeva S. Factors influencing quality of bowel preparation for colonoscopy. World Journal of Gastrointestinal Endoscopy. 2013;**5**(2):39-46. DOI: 10.4253/wjge.v5.i2.39

[14] Westerhof J, Koornstra JJ, Hoedemaker RA, Sluiter WJ, Kleibeuker JH, Weersma RK. Diagnostic yield of small bowel capsule endoscopy depends on the small bowel transit time. World Journal of Gastrointestinal Endoscopy. 2012;**18**(13):1502-1507. DOI: 10.3748/wjg.v18.i13.1502

[15] Rondonotti E, Pennazio M, Toth E, Koulaouzidis A. How to read small bowel capsule endoscopy: A practical guide for everyday use. Endoscopy International Open. 2020;**8**(10):E1220-E1224. DOI: 10.1055/a-1210-4830

[16] Koulaouzidis A, Dabos K, Philipper M, Toth E, Keuchel M. How should we do colon capsule endoscopy reading: A practical guide. Therapeutic Advances in Gastrointestinal Endoscopy. 2021;**14**:26317745211001983. DOI: 10.1177/26317745211001983

[17] Caunedo-Alvarez A, Romero-Vazquez J, Gomez-Rodriguez BJ, Sanchez-Yague A, Castro-Laria L, Herrerias-Gutierrez JM. Evaluation of a new double-headed biodegradable device (AGILE Patency Capsule) for detecting functional patency of the small intestine: A prospective clinical trial. In: Proceedings of the 5th International Conference on Capsule. Endoscopy. 2006

[18] Caunedo-Alvarez A, Romero-Vazquez J, Herrerias-Gutierrez JM. Patency and agile capsules. World Journal of Gastroenterology. 2008;**14**:5269-5273. DOI: 10.3748/wjg.14.5269

[19] Nemeth A, Kopylov U, Koulaouzidis A, et al. Use of patency capsule in patients with established Crohn's disease. Endoscopy. 2016;**48**:373-379

[20] Herrerias JM, Leighton JA, Costamagna G, Infantolino A, Eliakim R, Fischer D, et al. Agile patency system eliminates risk of capsule retention in patients with known intestinal strictures who undergo capsule endoscopy. Gastrointestinal Endoscopy. 2008;**67**:902-909. DOI: 10.1016/j.gie.2007.10.063

[21] Rezapour M, Amadi C, Gerson LB. Retention associated with video capsule endoscopy: Systematic review and meta-analysis. Gastrointestinal Endoscopy. 2017;**85**:1157-68.e2

[22] Gourtsoyiannis NC, Grammatikakis J, Papamastorakis G, et al. Imaging of small intestinal Crohn's disease: Comparison between MR enteroclysis and conventional enteroclysis. European Radiology. 2006;**16**:1915-1925

[23] Fork FT, Karlsson N, Kadhem S, et al. Small bowel enteroclysis with magnetic resonance imaging and computed tomography in patients with failed and uncertain passage of a patency capsule. BMC Medical Imaging. 2012;**12**:3

[24] Rozendorn N, Klang E, Lahat A. Prediction of patency capsule retention in known Crohn's disease patients by using magnetic resonance imaging. Gastrointestinal Endoscopy. 2016;**83**:182-187

[25] Spada C, Spera G, Riccioni M, et al. A novel diagnostic tool for detecting functional patency of the small bowel: The given patency capsule. Endoscopy. 2005;**37**:793-800

[26] Cohen SA, Gralnek IM, Ephrath H, et al. The use of a patency capsule in pediatric Crohn's disease: A prospective evaluation. Digestive Diseases and Sciences. 2011;**56**:860-865

[27] Peyrin-Biroulet L, Loftus EV Jr, Colombel JF, Sandborn WJ. The natural history of adult Crohn's disease

in population-based cohorts. The American Journal of Gastroenterology. 2010;**105**:289-297

[28] Thia KT, Sandborn WJ, Harmsen WS, Zinsmeister AR, Loftus EV Jr. Risk factors associated with progression to intestinal complications of Crohn's disease in a population-based cohort. Gastroenterology. 2010;**139**:1147-1155

[29] Tremaine WJ. Diagnosis and treatment of indeterminate colitis. Gastroenterology & Hepatology. 2011;**7**:826-828

[30] Zhou N, Chen WX, Chen SH, Xu CF, Li YM. Inflammatory bowel disease unclassified. Journal of Zhejiang University. Science. B. 2011;**12**:280-286

[31] Spada C, McNamara D, Despott EJ, Adler S, Cash BD, Fernández-Urién I, et al. Performance measures for small-bowel endoscopy: A European Society of Gastrointestinal Endoscopy (ESGE) quality improvement initiative. United European Gastroenterology Journal. 2019;**7**:614-641

[32] Agrawal M, Colombel JF. Treat-to-target in inflammatory bowel diseases, what is the target and how do we treat? Gastrointestinal Endoscopy Clinics of North America. 2019;**29**:421-436

[33] Peyrin-Biroulet L, Sandborn W, Sands BE, et al. Selecting therapeutic targets in inflammatory bowel disease (STRIDE): Determining therapeutic goals for treat-to-target. The American Journal of Gastroenterology. 2015;**110**:1324-1338

[34] Spada C, Hassan C, Galmiche JP, Neuhaus H, Dumonceau JM, Adler S, et al. Colon capsule endoscopy: European Society of Gastrointestinal Endoscopy (ESGE) guideline. Endoscopy. 2012;**44**(5):527-536

[35] Bourreille A, Ignjatovic A, Aabakken L, Loftus EV Jr, Eliakim R, Pennazio M, et al. Role of small-bowel endoscopy in the management of patients with inflammatory bowel disease: An international OMED-ECCO consensus. Endoscopy. 2009;**41**:618-637

[36] Juján-Sanchis M, Sanchis-Artero L, Larrey-Ruiz L, et al. Current role of capsule endoscopy in Crohn's disease. World Journal of Gastrointestinal Endoscopy. 2016;**8**:572-583

[37] Goran L, Negreanu AM, Stemate A, Negreanu L. Capsule endoscopy: Current status and role in Crohn's disease. World Journal of Gastrointestinal Endoscopy. 2018;**10**:184-192

[38] Papadakis KA, Tabibzadeh S. Diagnosis and misdiagnosis of inflammatory bowel disease. Gastrointestinal Endoscopy Clinics of North America. 2002;**12**:433-449. DOI: 10.1016/S1052-5157(02)00005-3

[39] Ng SC, Shi HY, Hamidi N, et al. Worldwide incidence and prevalence of inflammatory bowel disease in the 21st century: A systematic review of population-based studies. Lancet. 2017;**390**:2769-2778

[40] Torres J, Mehandru S, Colombel JF, Peyrin-Biroulet L. Crohn's disease. Lancet. 2017;**389**:1741-1755

[41] Van Hogezand RA, Witte AM, Veenendaal RA, Wagtmans MJ, Lamers CB. Proximal Crohn's disease: Review of the clinicopathologic features and therapy. Inflammatory Bowel Disease. 2001;**7**:328-337. DOI: 10.1097/00054725-200111000-00010

[42] Maaser C, Sturm A, Vavricka SR, Kucharzik T, Fiorino G, Annese V, et al. ECCO-ESGAR Guideline for Diagnostic

Assessment in IBD Part 1: Initial diagnosis, monitoring of known IBD, detection of complications. Journal of Crohn's and Colitis. 2019;**13**(2):144-164. DOI: 10.1093/ecco-jcc/jjy113

[43] Van Assche G, Dignass A, Panes J, et al. The second European evidence-based consensus on the diagnosis and management of Crohn's disease: Definitions and diagnosis. Journal of Crohn's & Colitis. 2010;**4**:7-27

[44] Lazarev M, Huang C, Bitton A, Cho JH, Duerr RH, McGovern DP, et al. Relationship between proximal Crohn's disease location and disease behavior and surgery: A cross-sectional study of the IBD genetics consortium. The American Journal of Gastroenterology. 2013;**108**:106-112

[45] Chow DK, Sung JJ, Wu JC, Tsoi KK, Leong RW, Chan FK. Upper gastrointestinal tract phenotype of Crohn's disease is associated with early surgery and further hospitalization. Inflammatory Bowel Diseases. 2009;**15**:551-557

[46] Levine A, Griffiths A, Markowitz J, Wilson DC, Turner D, Russell RK, et al. Pediatric modification of the Montreal classification for inflammatory bowel disease: The Paris classification. Inflammatory Bowel Diseases. 2011;**17**:1314-1321

[47] Mao R, Tang RH, Qiu Y, Chen BL, Guo J, Zhang SH, et al. Different clinical outcomes in Crohn's disease patients with esophagogastroduodenal, jejunal, and proximal ileal disease involvement: Is L4 truly a single phenotype? Therapeutic Advances in Gastroenterology. 2018;**11**:1756284818777938

[48] Jensen MD, Nathan T, Rafaelsen SR, Kjeldsen J. Diagnostic accuracy of capsule endoscopy for small bowel Crohn's disease is superior to that of MR enterography or CT enterography. Clinical Gastroenterology and Hepatology. 2011;**9**:124-129. DOI: 10.1016/j.cgh.2010.10.019

[49] Tillack C, Seiderer J, Brand S, Goke B, Reiser MF, Schaefer C, et al. Correlation of magnetic resonance enteroclysis (MRE) and wireless capsule endoscopy (CE) in the diagnosis of small bowel lesions in Crohn's disease. Inflammatory Bowel Diseases. 2008;**14**:1219-1228. DOI: 10.1002/ibd.20466

[50] Kharazmi AA, Aslani S, Kristiansen MF, Dahl EE, Berner-Hansen M. Indications and diagnostic yield of small-bowel capsule endoscopy in a real-world setting. BMC Gastroenterology. 2020;**20**:177. DOI: 10.1186/s12876-020-01326-8]

[51] Carretero C, Carbonnel F, Ferrante M, Knudsen T, Van Lent N, Lobo AJ, et al. Monitoring established Crohn's disease with pan-intestinal video capsule endoscopy in Europe: Clinician consultation using the nominal group technique. Current Medical Research and Opinion. 2021;**37**(9):1547-1554

[52] Pennazio M, Spada C, Eliakim R, et al. Small-bowel capsule endoscopy and device-assisted enteroscopy for diagnosis and treatment of small-bowel disorders: European Society of Gastrointestinal Endoscopy (ESGE) clinical guideline. Endoscopy. 2015;**47**:352-376

[53] Leighton JA, Legnani P, Seidman EG. Role of capsule endoscopy in inflammatory bowel disease: Where we are and where we are going. Inflammatory Bowel Diseases. 2007;**13**:331-337

[54] Girelli CM, Porta P, Malacrida V, Barzaghi F, Rocca F. Clinical outcome of

patients examined by capsule endoscopy for suspected small bowel Crohn's disease. Digestive and Liver Disease. 2007;**39**:148-154

[55] Hall B, Holleran G, Costigan D, McNamara D. Capsule endoscopy: High negative predictive value in the long term despite a low diagnostic yield in patients with suspected Crohn's disease. United European Gastroenterology Journal. 2013;**1**(6):461-466. DOI: 10.1177/2050640613508551

[56] Goldstein JL, Eisen GM, Lewis B, et al. Video capsule endoscopy to prospectively assess small bowel injury with celecoxib, naproxen plus omeprazole, and placebo. Clinical Gastroenterology and Hepatology. 2005;**3**:133-141

[57] Kumarasinghe MP, Quek TP, Chau CY, et al. Endoscopic biopsy features and diagnostic challenges of adult Crohn's disease at initial presentation. Pathology. 2010;**42**:131-137

[58] Mahadeva U, Martin JP, Patel NK, et al. Granulomatous ulcerative colitis: A re-appraisal of the mucosal granuloma in the distinction of Crohn's disease from ulcerative colitis. Histopathology. 2002;**41**:50-55

[59] Sakurai T, Saruta M. One study demonstrated that both FCP and CRP had low negative predictive values for small bowel where Pan-intestinal video capsule endoscopy (PCE) observed mucosal inflammation amongst patients with normal biomarker levels. Digestion. 2023;**104**:30-41

[60] Jung ES, Lee SP, Kae SH, Kim JH, Kim HS, Jang HJ. Diagnostic accuracy of fecal calprotectin for the detection of small bowel Crohn's disease through capsule endoscopy: An updated meta-analysis and systematic review. Gut Liver. 15 Sep 2021;**15**(5):732-741

[61] Koulaouzidis A, Douglas S, Rogers MA, Arnott ID, Plevris JN. Fecal calprotectin: A selection tool for small bowel capsule endoscopy in suspected IBD with prior negative bi-directional endoscopy. Scandinavian Journal of Gastroenterology. 2011;**46**(5):561-566. DOI: 10.3109/00365521.2011.551835

[62] Jones BH, Fleischer DE, Sharma VK, et al. Yield of repeat wireless video capsule endoscopy in patients with obscure gastrointestinal bleeding. The American Journal of Gastroenterology. 2005;**100**:1058-1064. DOI: 10.1111/j.1572-0241.2005.40722

[63] Viazis N, Papaxoinis K, Vlachogiannakos J, Efthymiou A, Theodoropoulos I, Karamanolis DG. Is there a role for second-look capsule endoscopy in patients with obscure GI bleeding after a nondiagnostic first test? Gastrointestinal Endoscopy. 2009;**69**(4):850-856

[64] Robertson AR, Yung DE, Arnott ID, Plevris JN. A Koulaouzidis capsule endoscopy in suspected small bowel Crohn's disease—Is it worth repeating a negative study? Digestive and Liver Disease. 2019;**51**(1):174-176. DOI: 10.1016/j.dld.2018.10.007

[65] Mielants H, De Keyser F, Baeten D, Van den Bosch F. Gut inflammation in the spondyloarthropathies. Current Rheumatology Reports. 2005;**7**:188-194

[66] Mielants H, Veys EM, Cuvelier C, De Vos M, Goemaere S, De Clerq L, et al. The evolution of spondylarthropathies in relation to gut histology: Part III. Prospective study of the clinical evolution of spondylarthropathies in relation to the evolution of gut histology. The Journal of Rheumatology. 1995;**22**:2279-2228

[67] Sagard J, Olofsson T, Mogard E, Marsal J, Andréasson K, Geijer M, et al.

Gut dysbiosis associated with worse disease activity and physical function in axial spondyloarthritis. Arthritis Research and Therapy. 2022;**24**:42

[68] Gracey E, Vereecke L, McGovern D, Fröhling M, Schett G, Danese S, et al. Revisiting the gut-joint axis: Links between gut inflammation and spondyloarthritis. Nature Reviews Rheumatology. 2020;**16**:415-433

[69] Kopylov U, Seidman EG. Diagnostic modalities for the evaluation of small bowel disorders. Current Opinion in Gastroenterology. 2015;**31**:111-117

[70] Eliakim R, Karban A, Markovits D, Bardan E, Bar-Meir S, Abramowich D, et al. Comparison of capsule endoscopy with ileocolonoscopy for detecting small-bowel lesions in patients with seronegative spondyloarthropathies. Endoscopy. 2005;**37**:1165-1169

[71] Hascelik G, Oz B, Olmez N, Memis A, Yoruk G, Unsal B, et al. Association of macroscopic gut inflammation with disease activity, functional status and quality of life in ankylosing spondylitis. Rheumatology International. 2009;**29**(7):755-758. DOI: 10.1007/s00296-008-0766-6

[72] Van Praet L, Van den Bosch FE, Jacques P, Carron P, Jans L, Colman R, et al. Microscopic gut inflammation in axial spondyloarthritis: A multiparametric predictive model. Annals of the Rheumatic Diseases. 2013;**72**:414-417

[73] Ben-Horin S, Lahat A, Amitai MM, et al. Assessment of small bowel mucosal healing by video capsule endoscopy for the prediction of short-term and longterm risk of Crohn's disease flare: A prospective cohort study. Lancet Gastroenterology & Hepatology. 2019;**4**(7):519-528. DOI: 10.1016/S2468-1253(19)30088

[74] Lorenzo-Zúñiga V, de Vega VM, Domènech E, Cabré E, Mañosa M, Boix J. Impact of capsule endoscopy findings in the management of Crohn's disease. Digestive Diseases and Sciences. 2010;**55**(2):411-414. DOI: 10.1007/s10620-009-0758-8

[75] Cotter J, Dias de Castro F, Moreira MJ, Rosa B. Tailoring Crohn's disease treatment: The impact of small bowel capsule endoscopy. Journal of Crohn's and Colitis. 2014;**8**(12):1610-1615. DOI: 10.1016/j.crohns.2014.02.018

[76] Leighton JA, Gralnek IM, Cohen SA, et al. Capsule endoscopy is superior to small-bowel follow-through and equivalent to ileocolonoscopy in suspected Crohn's disease. Clinical Gastroenterology and Hepatology. 2014;**12**:609-615

[77] Koulaouzidis A, Douglas S, Plevris JN. Lewis score correlates more closely with fecal calprotectin than capsule endoscopy Crohn's disease activity index. Digestive Diseases and Sciences. 2012;**57**:987-993

[78] Efthymiou A, Viazis N, Mantzaris G, et al. Does clinical response correlate with mucosal healing in patients with Crohn's disease of the small bowel? A prospective, case-series study using wireless capsule endoscopy. Inflammatory Bowel Diseases. 2008;**14**:1542-1547

[79] Niv E, Fishman S, Kachman H, et al. Sequential capsule endoscopy of the small bowel for follow-up of patients with known Crohn's disease. Journal of Crohn's & Colitis. Dec 2014;**8**(12):1616-1623. DOI: 10.1016/j.crohns.2014.03.003

[80] Bourreille A, Jarry M, D'Halluin PN, et al. Wireless capsule endoscopy versus ileocolonoscopy for the diagnosis of postoperative recurrence of Crohn's

disease: A prospective study. Gut. 2006;**55**:978-982

[81] Dubcenco E, Jeejeebhoy KN, Petroniene R, Tang S-j, Zalev AH, Gardiner GW, et al. Capsule endoscopy findings in patients with established and suspected small-bowel Crohn's disease: Correlation with radiologic, endoscopic, and histologic findings. Gastrointestinal Endoscopy. 2005;**62**(4):538-544. DOI: 10.1016/j.gie.2005.06.026

[82] Goran L, Negreanu AM, Stemate A, Negreanu L. Capsule endoscopy: Current status and role in Crohn's disease world. Journal of Gastrointestinal Endoscopy. 2018;**10**(9):184-192. DOI: 10.4253/wjge.v10.i9

[83] Hall B, Holleran G, Chin JL, Smith S, Ryan B, Mahmud N, et al. A prospective 52 week mucosal healing assessment of small bowel Crohn's disease as detected by capsule endoscopy. Journal of Crohn's & Colitis. 2014;**8**:1601-1609

[84] Shafran I, Burgunder P, DePanicis R, Fitch K, Hewit S, Abbott L. Evaluation of mucosal healing in small bowel Crohn's disease treated with certolizumab pegol assessed by wireless capsule endoscopy. Clinical Case Reports and Reviews. 2016;**2**(11):590-592. DOI: 10.15761/CCRR.1000284

[85] Kopylov U, Yablecovitch D, Lahat A, Neuman S, Levhar N, Greener T, et al. Detection of small bowel mucosal healing and deep remission in patients with known small bowel Crohn's disease using biomarkers, capsule endoscopy, and imaging. The American Journal of Gastroenterology. 2015;**110**:1316-1323

[86] Mitselos IV, Katsanos KH, Tatsioni A, Skamnelos A, Eliakim R, Tsianos EV, et al. Association of clinical and inflammatory markers with small bowel capsule endoscopy findings in Crohn's disease. European Journal of Gastroenterology & Hepatology. 2018;**30**:861-867

[87] Aggarwal V, Day AS, Connor S, Leach ST, Brown G, Singh R, et al. Role of capsule endoscopy and fecal biomarkers in small-bowel Crohn's disease to assess remission and predict relapse. Gastrointestinal Endoscopy. 2017;**86**:1070-1078

[88] Ma L, Li W, Zhuang N, Yang H, Liu W, Zhou W, et al. Comparison of transmural healing and mucosal healing as predictors of positive long-term outcomes in Crohn's disease. Therapeutic Advances in Gastroenterology. 2021;**14**:17562848211016259. DOI: 10.1177/17562848211016259

[89] Ben-Horin S, Lahat A, Amitai MM, Klang E, Yablecovitch D, Neuman S, et al. Assessment of small bowel mucosal healing by video capsule endoscopy for the prediction of short-term and long-term risk of Crohn's disease flare: A prospective cohort study. Lancet Gastroenterology & Hepatology. 2019;**4**(7):519-528. DOI: 10.1016/S2468-1253(19)30088-3

[90] Ooi CJ, Makharia GK, Hilmi I, Gibson PR, Fock KM, Ahuja V, et al. Asia Pacific consensus statements on Crohn's disease. Part 1: Definition, diagnosis, and epidemiology: (Asia Pacific Crohn's disease consensus—Part 1). Journal of Gastroenterology and Hepatology. 2016;**31**:45-55

[91] Triester SL, Leighton JA, Leontiadis GI, et al. A meta-analysis of the yield of capsule endoscopy compared to other diagnostic modalities in patients with non-stricturing small bowel Crohn's disease. The American Journal of Gastroenterology. 2006;**101**(5):954-964

[92] Leighton JA, Pasha SF. Inflammatory disorders of the small bowel. Gastrointestinal Endoscopy Clinics of North America. 2017;**27**(1):63-77. DOI: 10.1016/j.giec.2016.08.004

[93] Ou G, Enns R. Capsule endoscopy and small bowel Enteroscopy have they rendered the radiologist obsolete? Gastrointestinal Endoscopy Clinics of North America. 2019;**29**:471-485

[94] Lahat A, Kopylov U, Amitai MM, et al. Magnetic resonance enterography or video capsule endoscopy—what do Crohn's disease patients prefer? Patient Preference and Adherence. 2016;**10**:1043-1050

[95] Hansel SL, McCurdy JD, Barlow JM, et al. Clinical benefit of capsule endoscopy in Crohn's disease: Impact on patient management and prevalence of proximal small bowel involvement, Inflammatory Bowel Disease. 2018;**24**(7):1582-1588. DOI: 10.1093/ibd/izy050

[96] Adler SN, Yoav M, Eitan S, et al. Does capsule endoscopy have an added value in patients with perianal disease and a negative work up for Crohn's disease? World Journal of Gastrointestinal Endoscopy. 2012;**4**(5):185-188. DOI: 10.4253/wjge.v4.i5.185

[97] Melmed GY, Dubinsky MC, Rubin DT, et al. Utility of video capsule endoscopy for longitudinal monitoring of Crohn's disease activity in the small bowel: A prospective study. Gastrointestinal Endoscopy. 2018;**88**(6):947-955.e2. DOI: 10.1016/j.gie.2018.07.035

[98] Dionisio PM, Gurudu SR, Leighton JA, et al. Capsule endoscopy has a significantly higher diagnostic yield in patients with suspected and established small-bowel Crohn's disease: A meta-analysis. Am J Gastroenterol. 2010;**105**(6):1240-1248

[99] Kopylov U, Yung DE, Engel T, et al. Diagnostic yield of capsule endoscopy versus magnetic resonance enterography and small bowel contrast ultrasound in the evaluation of small bowel Crohn's disease: Systematic review and meta-analysis. Digestive and Liver Disease. Aug 2017;**49**(8):854-863. DOI: 10.1016/j.dld.2017.04.013

[100] Rondonotti E, Soncini M, Girelli C, et al. Small bowel capsule endoscopy in clinical practice: A multicenter 7-year survey. European Journal of Gastroenterology & Hepatology. 2010;**22**:1380-1386

[101] Fernández-Urién I, Carretero C, González B, et al. Incidence, clinical outcomes, and therapeutic approaches of capsule endoscopy-related adverse events in a large study population. Revista Española de Enfermedades Digestivas. 2015;**107**:745-752

[102] Palmer JS, Marenah K, El Madani F, Jain K, Gupta S. Small bowel perforation following capsule endoscopy: A case report. Annals of the Royal College of Surgeons of England. 2011;**93**:e69-e70. DOI: 10.1308/147870811X590829

[103] Skovsen AP, Burcharth J, Burgdorf SK. Capsule endoscopy: A cause of late small bowel obstruction and perforation. Case Rep Surg. 2013;**2013**:458108

[104] De Palma GD, Masone S, Persico M, et al. Capsule impaction presenting as acute small bowel perforation: A case series. Journal of Medical Case Reports. 2012;**6**:121

[105] Liao Z, Gao R, Xu C, Li ZS. Indications and detection, completion,

and retention rates of small-bowel capsule endoscopy: A systematic review. Gastrointestinal Endoscopy. 2010;**71**:280-286

[106] Nemeth A, Kopylov U, Koulaouzidis A, Wurm Johansson G, Thorlacius H, Amre D, et al. Use of patency capsule in patients with established Crohn's disease. Endoscopy. 2016;**48**(4):373-379. DOI: 10.1055/s-0034-1393560. Epub 2015 Nov 12. Patency capsule was shown to have a high false-positive rate (because of bowel motility)

[107] Rasmussen B, Nathan T, Jensen MD. Symptomatic patency capsule retention in suspected Crohn's disease. Journal of Crohn's & Colitis. 2016;**10**:1445-1447

[108] Rondonotti E, Herrrerias J, Pennazio M, et al. Complications, limitations, and failures of capsule endoscopy: A review of 733 cases. Gastrointestinal Endoscopy. 2005;**62**(5):712-716

[109] Ben-Soussan E, Savoye G, Antonietti M, et al. Factors that affect gastric passage of video capsule. Gastrointestinal Endoscopy. 2005;**62**(5):785-790

[110] Lucendo AJ, González-Castillo S, Fernández-Fuente M, De Rezende LC. Tracheal aspiration of a capsule endoscope: A new case report and literature compilation of an increasingly reported complication. Digestive Diseases and Sciences. 2011;**56**:2758-2762

[111] Mannami T et al. Capsule endoscope aspiration after repeated attempts for ingesting a patency capsule. Case Reports in Gastroenterology. 2015;**9**(3):347-335

[112] Fernández-Urién I et al. Incidence, clinical outcomes, and therapeutic approaches of capsule endoscopy-related adverse events in a large study population. Revista Espanola De Enfermedades Digestivas. 2015;**107**(12):745-752. DOI: 10.17235/reed.2015.3820/2015

[113] Wang Y-C, Pan J, Liu Y-W, Sun F-Y, Qian Y-Y, Jiang X, et al. Adverse events of video capsule endoscopy over the past two decades: A systematic review and proportion meta-analysis. BMC Gastroenterology. 2020;**20**:364. DOI: 10.1186/s12876-020-01491-w

[114] Lewis BS, Eisen GM, Friedman S. A pooled analysis to evaluate results of capsule endoscopy trials. Endoscopy. 2005;**37**:960-965. DOI: 10.1055/s-2005-870353

[115] Shamsudhin N, Zverev VI, Keller H, Pane S, Egolf PW, Nelson BJ, et al. Magnetically guided capsule endoscopy. Medical Physics. 2017;**44**:e91-e111. DOI: 10.1002/mp.12299

[116] Le Berre C, Sandborn WJ, Aridhi S, et al. Application of artificial intelligence to gastroenterology and hepatology. Gastroenterology. 2020;**158**(1):76-94.e2

[117] Pons BV, Nos P, Bastida G, Beltran B, Arguello L, Aguas M, et al. Evaluation of postsurgical recurrence in Crohn's disease: A new indication for capsule endoscopy? Gastrointestinal Endoscopy. 2007;**66**:533-540

[118] Rutgeerts P, Geboes K, Vantrappen G, Beyls J, Kerremans R, Hiele M. Predictability of the postoperative course of Crohn's disease. Gastroenterology. 1990;**99**:956-963

[119] Hammoudi N, Auzolle C, Tran Minh ML, et al. Postoperative endoscopic recurrence on the neoterminal ileum but not on the anastomosis is mainly driving long-term outcomes in Crohn's

disease. The American Journal of Gastroenterology. 2020;**115**(7):1084-1093

[120] Johnston C, Yung D, Joshi A, Plevris J, Koulaouzidis A. Small bowel malignancy in patients undergoing capsule endoscopy at a tertiary care academic center: Case series and review of the literature. Endoscopy International Open. 2017;**5**:463-470. DOI: 10.1055/s-0043-106186

[121] Kalla R, McAlindon ME, Drew K, Sidhu R. Clinical utility of capsule endoscopy in patients with Crohn's disease and inflammatory bowel disease unclassified. European Journal of Gastroenterology & Hepatology. 2013;**25**:706-713

[122] Min SB, Le-Carlson M, Singh N, Nylund CM, Gebbia J, Haas K, et al. Video capsule endoscopy impacts decision making in pediatric IBD: A single tertiary care center experience. Inflammatory Bowel Diseases. 2013;**19**:2139-2145

[123] Sara Monteiro X, de Castro FD, Carvalho PB, Rosa B, Moreira MJ, Pinho R, et al. Essential role of small bowel capsule endoscopy in reclassification of colonic inflammatory bowel disease type unclassified. World Journal of Gastrointestinal Endoscopy. 2017;**9**(1):34-40. DOI: 10.4253/wjge.v9.i1.34

[124] Yung DE, Rondonotti E, Giannakou A, Avni T, Rosa B, Toth E, et al. Capsule endoscopy in young patients with iron deficiency anaemia and negative bidirectional gastrointestinal endoscopy. United European Gastroenterol J. 2017;**5**(7):974-981. DOI: 10.1177/2050640617692501

[125] Niv Y, Ilani S, Levi Z, Hershkowitz M, Niv E, Fireman Z, et al. Validation of the capsule endoscopy Crohn's disease activity index (CECDAI or Niv score): A multicenter prospective study. Endoscopy. 2012;**44**(1):21-26. DOI: 10.1055/s-0031-1291385

[126] Gralnek IM, Defranchis R, Seidman E, Leighton JA, Legnani P, Lewis BS. Development of a capsule endoscopy scoring index for small bowel mucosal inflammatory change. Alimentary Pharmacology & Therapeutics. 2008;**27**:146-154

[127] Tukey M, Pleskow D, Legnani P, et al. The utility of capsule endoscopy in patients with suspected Crohn's disease. The American Journal of Gastroenterology. 2009;**104**:2734-2739

[128] Figueiredo P, Almeida N, Lopes S, et al. Small-bowel capsule endoscopy in patients with suspected Crohn's disease-diagnostic value and complications. Diagnostic and Therapeutic Endoscopy. 2010;**2010**. pii: 101284

[129] Na SY, Lim YJ. Capsule endoscopy in inflammatory bowel disease: When? To whom? Diagnostics (Basel). 2021;**11**(12):2240. DOI: 10.3390/diagnostics11122240

[130] Hwang Y, Park J, Lim YJ, Chun HJ. Application of artificial intelligence in capsule endoscopy: Where are we now? Clinical Endoscopy. 2018;**51**(6):547-551. DOI: 10.5946/ce.2018.173

[131] Saraiva MM, Ferreira JPS, Cardoso H, Afonso J, Ribeiro T, Andrade P, et al. Artificial intelligence and colon capsule endoscopy: Development of an automated diagnostic system of protruding lesions in colon capsule endoscopy. Techniques in Coloproctology. 2021;**25**:1243-1248

[132] Klang E, Barash Y, Margalit RY, et al. Deep learning algorithms for automated detection of Crohn's disease

ulcers by video capsule endoscopy. Gastrointestinal Endoscopy. 2020;**91**:606.e2-613.e2

[133] Mascarenhas Saraiva MJ, Afonso J, Ribeiro T, et al. Deep learning and capsule endoscopy: Automatic identification and differentiation of small bowel lesions with distinct haemorrhagic potential using a convolutional neural network. BMJ Open Gastroenterology. 2021;**8**:e000753

[134] Souchaud M, Houist G, et al. A neural network-based algorithm for assessing the cleanliness of small bowel during capsule endoscopy. Endoscopy. 2021;**53**:932-936

[135] Langlotz CP, Allen B, Erickson BJ, et al. A roadmap for foundational research on artificial intelligence in medical imaging: From the 2018 nih/rsna/acr/the academy workshop. Radiology. 2019;**291**:781-791

[136] Herp J, Deding U, Buijs MM, Kroijer R, Baatrup G, Nadimi ES. Feature point tracking-based localization of Colon capsule endoscope. Diagnostics. 2021;**11**:193

[137] Muehlematter UJ, Daniore P, Vokinger KN. Approval of artificial intelligence and machine learning-based medical devices in the USA and Europe (2015-20): A comparative analysis. Lancet Digital Health. 2021;**3**:e195-e203. DOI: 10.1016/S2589-7500(20)30292-2)

[138] McCain JD, Pasha SF, Leighton JA. Role of capsule endoscopy in inflammatory bowel disease. Gastrointestinal Endoscopy Clinics of North America. 2021;**31**:34

Chapter 5

Endoscopic Management of Fistulas and Abscesses in Crohn's Disease

Partha Pal, Rupa Banerjee, Mohan Ramchandani, Rajendra Patel, Zaheer Nabi, Swathi Kanaganti, Rajesh Gupta, Manu Tandan and Duvvuru Nageshwar Reddy

Abstract

Fistulas and abscesses in Crohn's disease (CD) are mechanical complications of long term disease and can indicate an aggressive disease course. Usually chronic inflammation leads to stricture which leads to high intra-luminal pressure with resultant fistula and abscess upstream to stricture. Exceptions to that may include perianal fistulizing CD which may even precede luminal CD. Hence, management of fistula and abscesses entails management of associated strictures without which these are bound to recur. These mechanical complications (stricture/fistula/abscess) usually occur after initial 4–5 years of disease. Traditionally the management of these complications include surgical therapy. However, surgical therapy can be associated with substantial morbidity specially in these patients on immunosuppressive medications and post-operative recurrence is not uncommon. Interventional radiological procedures to drain intra-abdominal/pelvic abscess can be helpful provided that there are no intervening bowel loops. Hence, there is an unmet need of relatively less invasive endoscopic therapies for treatment of CD related fistulas and abscesses. In this chapter, we shall discuss the role of endoscopic therapy in CD related fistula and abscess.

Keywords: Crohn's disease, fistulotomy, seton, glue, plug, over the scope clips, drainage, endoscopic ultrasound

1. Introduction

Endoscopic treatment of fistula initially includes initial treatment of associated stricture (with endoscopic balloon dilation/stricturotomy or self expanding metal stents-SEMS) and drainage of abscess if any [1]. Chronic fistula are usually the result of transmural disease and fibrosis and hence should usually be treated with opening up of the fistula rather than closure which can be done for acute leaks. The treatment modalities include opening up the fistula by cutting (fistulotomy), filling the fistula with fistula plug/glue injection/stem cell injection or fistula closure with SEMS/endoscopic suturing/clipping [2]. However, the knowledge of underlying pathology and patient selection are important for such procedures to increase the overall success rate. Usually, short, superficial, simple, bowel to bowel fistulas were ideal for endoscopic therapy. On the contrary, endoscopic therapy for long, deep fistulas close to anal sphincters and anterior rectal walls (due to close proximity to genital structures) are better avoided.

2. Patient selection for endoscopic therapy for fistula in Crohn's disease

Fistulas in Crohn's disease are diagnosed based on clinical, radiologic and endoscopic findings. External fistulas consists of nearly two-third of all CD related fistulas. Among them, the majority are peri-anal fistulas whereas minority are enterocutaneous fistulas. Internal fistulas (nearly one third of all fistulas) consist of enteroenteric and rectovaginal fistulas. As mentioned earlier, patient selection is the key to success for endoscopic therapy for CD related fistulas. The length, depth, complexity, concurrent inflammation and organs involved in the feeding/exiting side of the fistula influence the patient selection. Bowel to bowel fistula are appropriate for endoscopic therapy, whereas extreme caution should be exercised for enterocutaneous fistula. CD related de novo fistula and those from gut to hollow organs (bladder, vagina) should be treated with surgery. Short (<3 cm), shallow (<2 cm deep), benign and non-complex fistulas are ideal for endoscopic therapy (**Figure 1**) [2].

3. Steps of endoscopic management of CD related fistula

The first step of treating CD related fistula is to drain associated abscess or treat associated stricture. All these fistula has a feeding side on the bowel side from which

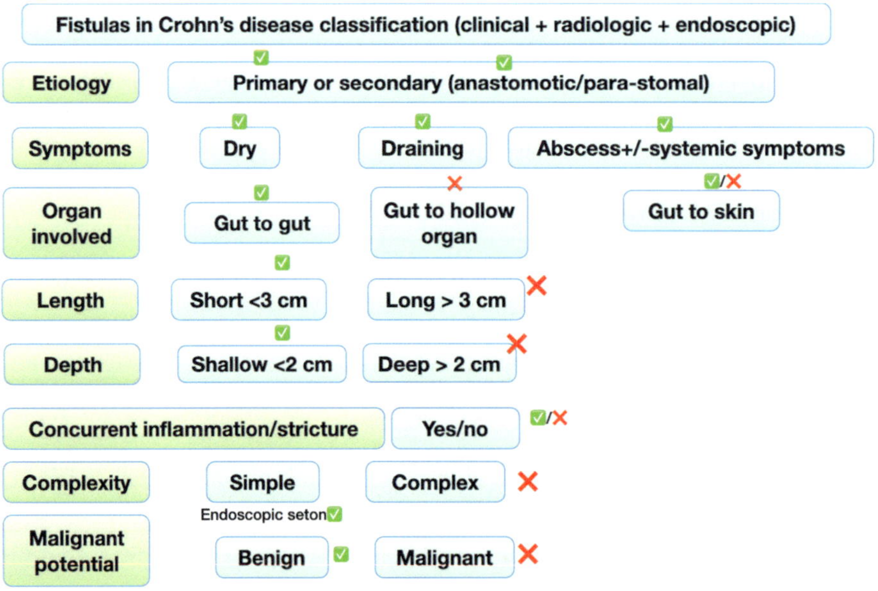

Figure 1.
Patient selection for endoscopic therapy in Crohn's disease based on classification of fistulas. Tick marks (√) indicate feasibility of endoscopic therapy whereas cross marks (X) indicate that endoscopic therapy is not feasible. Both tick and cross mark indicate the need for caution in these settings.

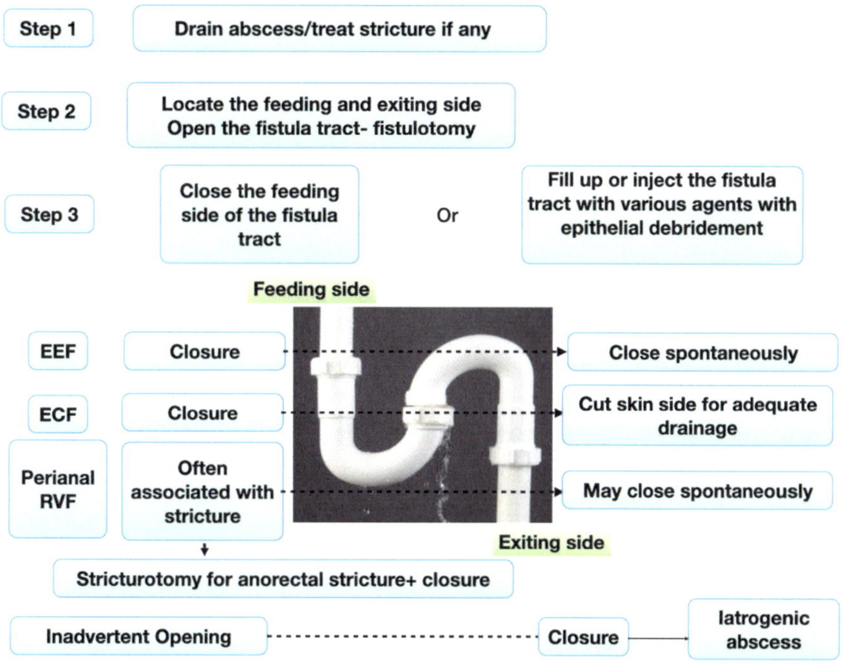

Figure 2.
Steps of endoscopic management of Crohn's disease related fistulas. EEF: Entero-enteric fistula, ECF-enterocutaneous fistula, RVF-rectovaginal fistula.

there is flow of bowel contents to existing site which can be bowel/skin or a hollow organ. In the second step, these sides should be located. Fistulotomy can be done for chronic fistulas. Feeding side can be closed in the third step with filling up of fistula tract with various sclerosing agents/plugs. The exiting side closes spontaneously after closure of feeding side in enter-enteric fistula. Closure of the feeding side of enterocutaneous fistula needs additional opening up on the exiting side for adequate drainage. Perianal and rectovaginal fistulas are often assisted with stricture which should be treated followed by closure of feeding side. Associated stricture and abscess can be treated endoscopically with endoscopic balloon dilation/endoscopic stricturotomy/stenting and endoscopic incision and drainage by needle knife/seton placement/endoscopic ultrasound (EUS) guided drainage of pelvic abscess (specially if overlying bowel loops hinder radiological drainage). Exiting side usually closes spontaneously in these circumstances. Inadvertent opening of feeding side or closure of exiting side can lead to iatrogenic abscess (**Figure 2**) [2].

4. Endoscopic drainage of abscess

Endoscopic drainage of CD related abscess can be done for perianal abscess or pelvic abscess. Complete drainage for perianal fistula can be done by short, superficial fistula outside external anal sphincter using needle knife (**Figure 3**). Partial drainage can be helpful in long fistulas close to the anal sphincter [2]. Pelvic abscess in close proximity to rectal wall can be drained by endoscopic ultrasound (EUS) guided single time aspiration or pigtail stent drainage. Cases in which interventional radiology is not feasible due to overlying bowel, EUS guided drainage can be particularly helpful (**Figure 4**) [2].

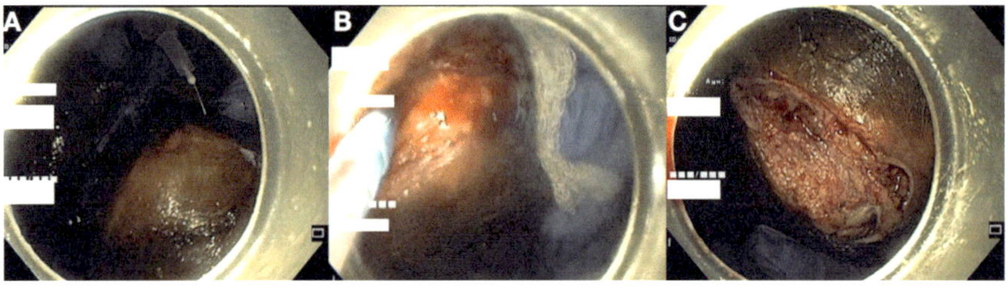

Figure 3.
Endoscopic perianal abscess drainage. A. Recurrent peri-anal abscess post surgical fistulotomy and seton placement, B. Fistulotomy along previous surgical fistulotomy line with needle knife, C. Post endoscopic fistulotomy.

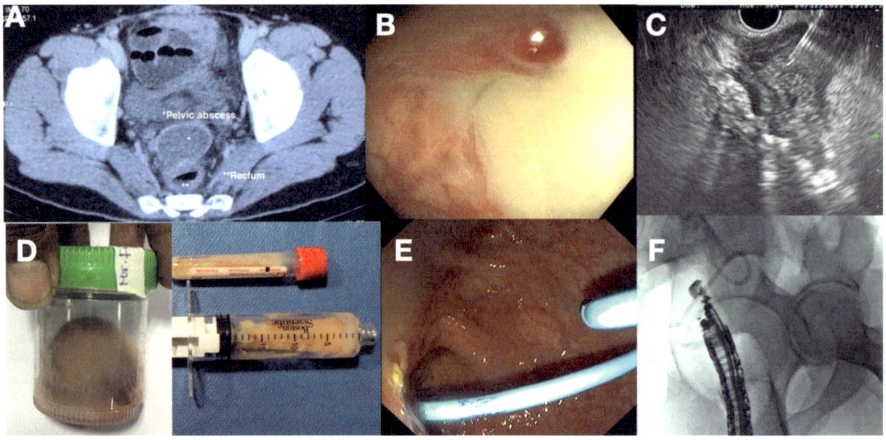

Figure 4.
Endoscopic ultrasound (EUS) guided drainage of pelvic abscess. A. Computed tomography shows pelvic abscess anterior to anterior rectal wall, B. Pus draining from fistulous opening on colonoscopy, C. EUS guided puncture and aspiration of pelvic abscess using 19 G fine needle aspiration needle, D. Aspirated pus, E. Pigtail stent placed under EUS guidance after tract dilation with 6 Fr cystotome, F. Fluoroscopy showing echoendoscope and pigtail stent.

5. Endoscopic seton placement

Endoscopic seton placement can be done for short, superficial perianal fistulas in which internal opening is located close to anal verge and external opening is located nearby in perianal area. The internal opening can be located under endoscopic guidance or by injection of hydrogen peroxide/dye (e.g., indigo carmine/methylene blue) through external opening. Once located, a flexible soft tip guidewire (e.g., Jag wire) can be introduced through the external opening to pass it through the internal opening. This may not be feasible in complex, long, branching fistulas. Once, the guidewire is passed through internal opening, it can be grasped by forceps under endoscopic guidance and a draining seton can be tied over the guidewire. The guidewire is then pulled to place the seton across the fistula following which multiple knots should be applied to prevent early migration of seton (**Figure 5**). Endoscopic seton placement is particularly helpful in CD related simple fistula or re-introduction of seton in case of prior surgical placement of seton.

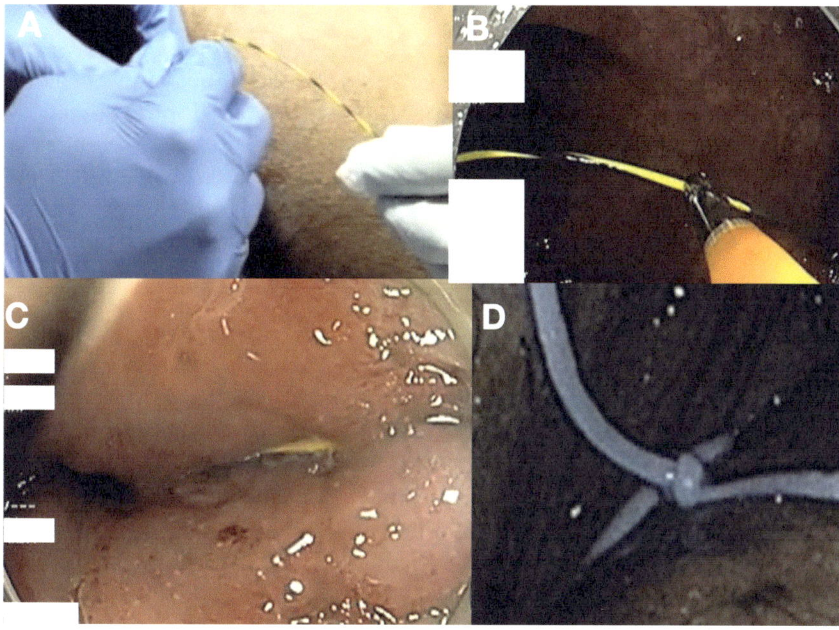

Figure 5.
Endoscopic seton placement. A. Guidewire passed through external fistula opening, B. Guidewire grabbed with forceps once it came out of internal opening, C. Guidewire seen coming out of internal opening located at anal verge. D. Endoscopic seton placed.

6. Endoscopic fistulotomy

Endoscopic fistulotomy in IBD can be done for exiting side of perianal fistula, primary ileo-cecal fistula and postoperative bowel-bowel fistula at suture line or anastomotic site. The largest case series till date (n = 29) have described the feasibility of fistulotomy mainly in pouch related fistulas (n = 21) although fistulotomy has been described for perianal fistula (n-6) and fistula from ileo-colonic anastomotic site to colon [3]. Fistula resolution and clinical success were reported in 89.6 and 75.8%, respectively. Bleeding was described in one case and no cases of perforation was reported [3]. Fistulotomy for enterocutaneous fistula is limited to case reports [4]. After fistulotomy, additional endoclips can prevent re-approximation of the fistula tract. Fistulotomy is an option for short and shallow fistulas.

7. Injection of filling materials

7.1 Glue

After seton removal, glue injection can lead to better (38%) anal fistula healing compared to observation alone (16%) as shown in a randomized controlled trial (RCT) [5]. In a retrospective study of 119 patients, fibrin glue injection led to complete fistula remission in 45.4% at 1 year. Higher fistula healing (63%) was seen in those on combined biologic and immunomodulator therapy [6]. Fibrin glue as an adjunctive therapy with anal advancement flap for repair of complex anal fistula showed no definite benefit over anal advancement flap alone as shown in a RCT [7].

7.2 Anal fistula plug (AFP)

AFP placement can be done under endoscopic guidance although it is usually placed in the operating theater by surgeons. The results of AFP for CD related fistulas are conflicting. In contrast to glue injection, AFP was not useful after seton removal compared to observation alone for anorectal fistula according to a RCT [8]. A prospective study showed high success rates (80% of patients: n = 20; 83% among fistula tracts: n = 36) specially for simple fistula. A long term follow up study with a median follow up 110 months showed a lower overall healing rate (38%). No incremental benefit was seen after placement of three fistula plugs [9].

7.3 Stem cells

Studies evaluating stem cell injection for CD related fistula have done it surgically although such injections can be easily done under endoscopic guidance. In CD related refractory, complex fistula, adipose tissue derived allogenic stem cell injection (120 million cells) have shown to be effective in inducing clinical and radiologic remission at 24 weeks (51 vs. 36% placebo) followed by maintaining remission at 52 weeks (56.3 vs. 38.6% placebo) [10, 11].

7.4 Sclerosing agents

Repeated injections (n = 3) of 50% dextrose and doxycycline have been shown to induce fibrosis and facilitate healing in pouch related fistulas although it can be tried in other CD related fistulas as well [12].

8. Endoscopic closure

8.1 Endoscopic clipping

CD related fistula are results of transmural bowel inflammation and hence endoscopic clipping is not very effective in CD related chronic or primary/de novo fistula closure. However, over the scope clips (OTSC) can be useful for acute post surgical leaks/perforations with single tract and minimal/no inflammation [2]. Through the scope (TTS) clips designed for bleeding control are ineffective for CD related fistulas. Case series have shown 70% technical success rate with OTSC [13]. OTSC should not be used for bowel to hollow organ fistula (rectovaginal) due to suboptimal success and risk of fistula worsening due to thin septum between rectum and vagina. OTSC for closure of intestinal side of enterocutaneous fistula can be done but extreme caution should be exercised and the skin side should be adequately drained [13]. But it should be kept in mind that the results are not very encouraging and there is limited data.

Fistula endoscopic submucosal dissection (ESD) with OTSC closure have been described for non-IBD refractory fistulas. There is no literature on CD related fistula.

8.2 Endoscopic suturing

Endoscopic suturing as a closure method have not been described for IBD fistulas but it can be technically feasible in distal bowel. It should not be attempted in bowel to hollow organ fistulas (recto-vaginal) and proximal bowel fistulas (technically difficult) [2]. However, suturing can be used for large perforations as a complication of endoscopic therapy or SEMS fixation.

8.3 Endoscopic stenting

The long term efficacy of FCSEMS for CD related fistula is unknown and evidence is limited to case series [14]. Stent fixation is mandatory to prevent migration in the absence of associated stricture.

9. Conclusion

Endoscopic therapy for fistulas and abscesses (**Figure 6**) in CD is challenging due to chronic, transmural nature of disease with high risk of complications due to diseased bowel, poor nutrition and concurrent immunosuppressant use. However, these therapies can delay or prevent surgery, act as an adjunct or help manage post-operative complications. There are paucity of prospective, controlled trials supporting endoscopic therapy for CD related fistula and abscess and are mostly limited to case-series/reports and retrospective studies. Future multi-centre, prospective, comparative studies with can help positioning of these novel approaches in the management algorithm of CD reacted fistulas.

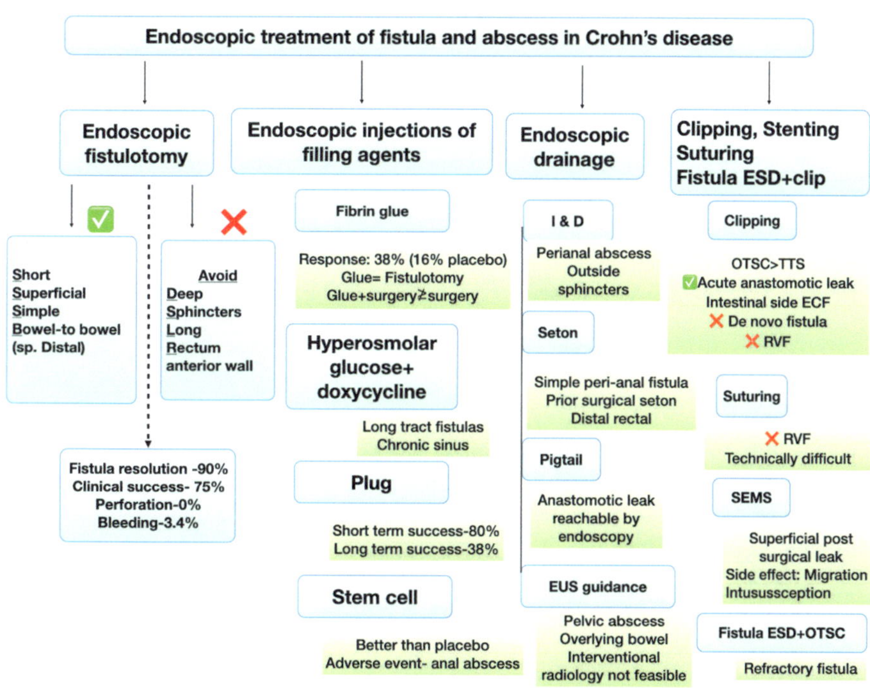

Figure 6.
Summary of endoscopic therapy for Crohn's disease related fistulas. I&D: Incision and drainage, OTSC-over the scope clips, TTS-through the scope clips, RVF-rectovaginal fistula, SEMS-self expanding meta stents, ESD-endoscopic submucosal dissection, ECF-enterocutaneous fistula. (√) indicate feasibility of endoscopic fistulotomy whereas cross marks (X) indicate that endoscopic fistulotomy is not feasible.

Authors' contribution

Conceptualization: PP; Literature review and writing original draft: PP, SK, Illustrations: PP; proof reading and critical review: MT, RG, RP, RB, MR, DNR, approving final manuscript: PP, SK, RB, MR, RP, RG, DNR, MT.

Conflict of interest

None.

Guarantor of the article

Partha Pal.

Financial disclosure

None.

Author details

Partha Pal*, Rupa Banerjee, Mohan Ramchandani, Rajendra Patel, Zaheer Nabi, Swathi Kanaganti, Rajesh Gupta, Manu Tandan and Duvvuru Nageshwar Reddy
Department of Medical Gastroenterology, Asian Institute of Gastroenterology, Hyderabad, Telangana, India

*Address all correspondence to: partha0123456789@gmail.com

References

[1] Cosnes J, Cattan S, Blain A, Beaugerie L, Carbonnel F, Parc R, et al. Long-term evolution of disease behavior of Crohn's disease. Inflammatory Bowel Diseases. 2002;**8**(4):244-250

[2] Lan N, Shen B. Endoscopic therapy for fistulas and abscesses in Crohn's disease. Gastrointestinal Endoscopy Clinics of North America. 2022;**32**(4):733-746

[3] Kochhar G, Shen B. Endoscopic fistulotomy in inflammatory bowel disease (with video). Gastrointestinal Endoscopy. 2018;**88**(1):87-94

[4] Lee H, Shen B. Endoscopic Fistulotomy heals a Y-shaped enterocutaneous fistula. ACG Case Reports Journal. 2017;**4**:e60

[5] Grimaud JC, Munoz-Bongrand N, Siproudhis L, Abramowitz L, Sénéjoux A, Vitton V, et al. Fibrin glue is effective healing perianal fistulas in patients with Crohn's disease. Gastroenterology. 2010;**138**(7): 2275-2281 81.e1

[6] Vidon M, Munoz-Bongrand N, Lambert J, Maggiori L, Zeitoun JD, Corte H, et al. Long-term efficacy of fibrin glue injection for perianal fistulas in patients with Crohn's disease. Colorectal Disease. 2021;**23**(4):894-900

[7] Ellis CN, Clark S. Fibrin glue as an adjunct to flap repair of anal fistulas: A randomized, controlled study. Diseases of the Colon and Rectum. 2006;**49**(11):1736-1740

[8] Senéjoux A, Siproudhis L, Abramowitz L, Munoz-Bongrand N, Desseaux K, Bouguen G, et al. Fistula plug in fistulising ano-perineal Crohn's disease: A randomised controlled trial. Journal of Crohn's & Colitis. 2016;**10**(2):141-148

[9] Aho Fält U, Zawadzki A, Starck M, Bohe M, Johnson LB. Long-term outcome of the Surgisis(®) (biodesign(®)) anal fistula plug for complex cryptoglandular and Crohn's fistulas. Colorectal Disease. 2021;**23**(1):178-185

[10] Panés J, García-Olmo D, Van Assche G, Colombel JF, Reinisch W, Baumgart DC, et al. Expanded allogeneic adipose-derived mesenchymal stem cells (Cx601) for complex perianal fistulas in Crohn's disease: A phase 3 randomised, double-blind controlled trial. Lancet. 2016;**388**(10051):1281-1290

[11] Panés J, García-Olmo D, Van Assche G, Colombel JF, Reinisch W, Baumgart DC, et al. Long-term efficacy and safety of stem cell therapy (Cx601) for complex perianal fistulas in patients with Crohn's disease. Gastroenterology. 2018;**154**(5):1334-42.e4

[12] Nyabanga CT, Obusez EC, Purysko A, Shen B. Healing of a chronic anal stump sinus after administration of combined high-concentration dextrose and doxycycline solution. International Journal of Colorectal Disease. 2016;**31**(3):775-776

[13] Mennigen R, Laukötter M, Senninger N, Rijcken E. The OTSC(®) proctology clip system for the closure of refractory anal fistulas. Techniques in Coloproctology. 2015;**19**(4):241-246

[14] Cereatti F, Fiocca F, Dumont JL, Ceci V, Vergeau BM, Tuszynski T, et al. Fully covered self-expandable metal stent in the treatment of postsurgical colorectal diseases: Outcome in 29 patients. Therapeutic Advances in Gastroenterology. 2016;**9**(2):180-188